COPYCAT RECIPES COOKBOOK

More Than 250 Recipes From The Most Famous Restaurants Around The World! Never Have To Worry How To Surprise Your Friends And Familiars With These Easy And Quick Dishes!

By
Brenda Loss

TABLE OF CONTENTS

INTRODUCTION

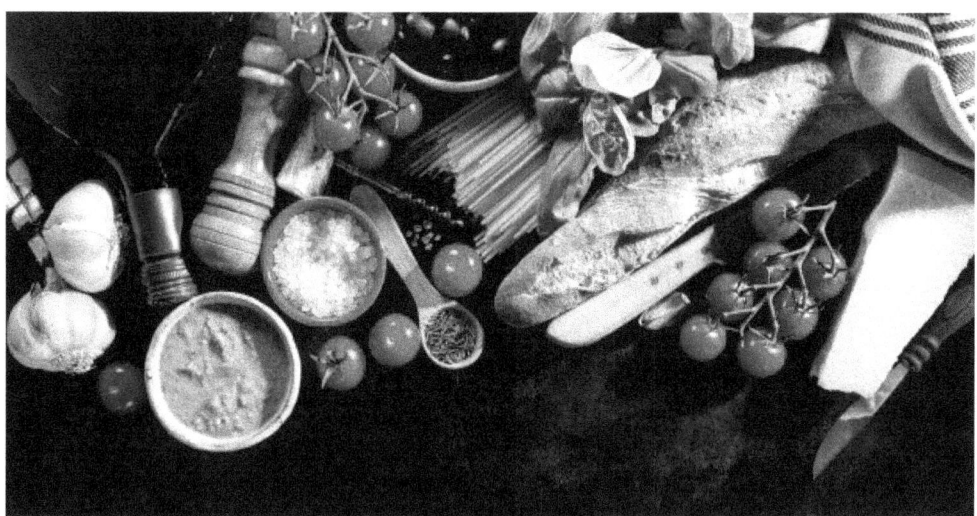

*A*ll these recipes use basic ingredients that can be found in any grocery store. It is not really that difficult to learn how to cook top-secret restaurant recipes. Some think you need a degree in culinary arts or cooking education so you can cook those secret recipes. I hate telling you this, but anyone can collect the ingredients themselves and cook a fancy meal that tastes like the real thing. Here, you will find tips on how to create the restaurant feeling at home. You'll get a list of basic cookware and appliances you need to have in your kitchen as well as how to stock your pantry to prepare some amazing dishes. There will be a primer on how to choose the best and freshest ingredients. You will also learn the basic cooking terms and techniques used in here. Copycat restaurant recipes are now widely known because of the ever-high cost of eating out. These copycat restaurant recipes are the hidden recipes from all your favorite restaurants in America so you can prepare them in the comfort of your home. The benefit of using copycat restaurant recipes is that not only can you save money; you can also customize the recipes. For example, if you want to reduce the salt or butter in one of the plates, you can. Now you've saved money, and at the same time provided a nutritious meal for your family. You have little control over the ingredients in the meal when you eat out. You can't, of course, adjust the dish that you order because sauces, etc. are made in advance. All of us know that it is expensive to take our family out for dinner, and without a doubt, this would easily cost you around a hundred dollars on an average. With copycat restaurant recipes the same one hundred dollars can easily produce 4 or more meals. Having regular meals inspired *by your favorite restaurants as a family allows for a healthier, more tight-knit family. Research have shown that, families who dine together at home are more united, and the kids perform better. Cooking recipes copied from restaurants will also amaze your friends and family who will ask themselves << where did you learn to cook so well ? >>. Imagine cooking a whole meal that appears to be the restaurant's takeaway food. I bet some of your friends won't even believe you cooked it!*

BREAKFAST RECIPES

Denny's French toast

Servings: 6-8 portions

Nutrition: Carbohydrates 33g /Protein 10g /Fat 17g

Ingredients:

- 4 eggs
- 2⁄3 cup whole milk
- 1⁄3 cup flour
- 1⁄3 cup sugar
- 1⁄2 teaspoon vanilla
- 1⁄4 teaspoon salt
- 1⁄8 teaspoon cinnamon
- 6 slices Texas toast thick bread
- 3 tablespoons butter
- powdered sugar
- butter
- syrup

Instructions:

1. Mix collectively the eggs, milk, flour, sugar, vanilla, salt& cinnamon.

2. Heat a massive skillet, or griddle.

3. When the skillet is hot, add 1 tablespoon butter.

4. If the butter smokes, your pan is simply too warm; flip down the warmth.

5. Dip each slice of bread into the batter for 30 seconds on every side.

6. Let a number of the batter drip off, then installed skillet.

7. Cook each slice 1 1/2-2 minutes in step with facet till every aspect is golden brown.

8. Add extra butter, if necessary, to cook dinner all of the slices.

9. To serve, put on plate, dirt with powdered sugar. Serve with butter & hot syrup.

IHOP "Harvest Grain 'N Nut" pancakes

Servings: 10 pancakes

Nutrition: Carbohydrates: 30g /Protein: 7g /Fat: 5g

Ingredients:

- 1 1/2 cup quick oats - 1 1/2 cups whole wheat flour
- 2 tsp baking soda - 1 tsp baking powder
- 1/4 tsp salt
- 1/4 cup unsweetened applesauce
- 1 3/4 cups
- 1 1/2 tsp white vinegar
- 4 tbsp brown sugar
- 2 egg whites
- 3 tbsp finely chopped walnuts
- 3 tbsp finely chopped blanched almonds
- 1 cup of milk

Instructions:

1. Mix milk and vinegar together and set aside.

2. Grind the oats in a blender or food processor till fine. In a big bowl, combine floor oats, entire wheat flour, baking soda, baking powder, and salt.

3. Beat the egg whites in a separate bowl till stiff peaks form.

4. In every other bowl, combine, milk blended with vinegar, applesauce and sugar with an electric powered mixer till smooth.

5. Finely chop walnuts and almonds and stir into aggregate. Fold in whipped egg whites

6. Lightly oil a skillet or griddle, and preheat it to medium warmth.

Ladle half of cup of the batter onto the hot skillet.

7. Cook the pancakes for two to four mins consistent with side, or till brown. Flip when the surface simply starts to bubble.

8. I use a skinny spatula - I discover it simpler to turn the pancakes with one like this.

9. If the mixture starts to thicken an excessive amount of upload touch milk (1-2 tsp till the consistency is returned to how it turned into initially)

10. Garnish with Apple Cinnamon topping and mild whipped cream, extra cinnamon, and nuts, if desired.

McDonald's Sausage Egg McMuffin

Servings : 4 servings

Nutrition: Carbohydrates: 67.3g/ Protein: 14.6g / Fat: 14.9g

Ingredients:

Sausage Patties

- 1 lb / 500g ground pork (juicier) OR beef (mince) (Note 1)
- 1/2 tsp dried ground sage
- 1/2 tsp dried thyme
- 1 tsp onion powder (or garlic powder)
- 3/4 tsp black pepper
- 3/4 tsp salt
- 1/2 tsp sugar (any)

Muffins

- 2 tbsp oil - 4 eggs
- 4 English muffins , cut in half
- 4 slices cheese

Instructions:

1. Preheat oven to 130C/275F.

2. Place muffins on a baking tray, cut side up, and pinnacle with cheese. (Alternative - soften cheese on sausage patties)

3. Mix Sausage Patty elements in a bowl - use your hands to combine it actual good.!

4. Shape.into 4 patties (thick ones, or 5 Maccers length patties).

5. Heat oil in a big nonstick skillet over high warmth. Add patties (in batches if needed). Cook the first side for 2 - 3 minutes or until browned. Flip then cook dinner the alternative side till browned.

6. Meanwhile, warmth any other pan over medium-high warmth with 1 tbsp oil. Spray egg rings with oil and area inside the skillet.

7. Crack egg into the rings. Add around 2 tbsp water into the skillet then cowl with a lid. Cook for 1 - 2 minutes or till egg is cooked for your liking.

8. Remove warm desserts from the oven. Top with sausage, then egg, the lid of muffin.

9. Serve and enjoy!

Starbucks Spinach and feta breakfast rolls Servings
Serving: 1 servings

Nutrition: Carbohydrates: 42g /Protein: 24g /Fat: 14g

Ingredients:

- 3 large egg whites
- 1/4 teaspoon ground turmeric
- 1/8 teaspoon ground black pepper cooking spray
- 2 cups spinach, chopped
- 1 medium tomato, insides scooped out and remainder finely chopped
- 1 burrito-size whole wheat tortilla (10 inches across)
- 1 tablespoon plain low-fat cream cheese
- 2 tablespoons crumbled feta cheese

Instructions:

1. In a small bowl, whisk collectively egg whites, black pepper, and turmeric.

2. Coat a medium pan with a light layer of cooking spray, over medium warmth. Add the eggs and let cook until the bottom sets, approximately two mins. Flip to cook dinner the alternative side, about half a minute, then take away from pan.

3. Coat the pan with a mild layer of cooking spray again, if needed. Add spinach to one facet and tomato to the opposite. Let cook dinner, retaining separate and occasionally stirring till spinach is barely wilted (approximately two mins), and tomatoes are cooked (about 4 minutes). Remove from pan.

4. Spread out your tortilla on a large plate or cutting board.

5. Spread at the cream cheese, leaving about an inch empty on all sides of the tortilla, then sprinkle the feta cheese on top.

6. Arrange spinach and tomatoes over the feta.

7. Fold the eggs into three and vicinity toward one facet of the tortilla. Fold over the top and bottom of the tortilla in the direction of the middle, then fold over the eggs in the direction of the center and preserve rolling tightly until you reach the alternative end.

8. Return the wrap to the pan, seam facet down. Heat over medium for three mins on every facet, till crisped up and golden brown. Cut in 1/2 and serve.

Jimmy Dean's homemade pork sausage

Servings: 3 servings

Nutrition: Carbohydrates: 2g/ Protein: 9g/ Fat: 19g

Ingredients:

- Pork
- Water
- Pork Broth
- Corn Syrup
- Salt
- Spices
- Vinegar
- Sugar
- Monosodium Glutamate
- Spice Extractives
- Natural Flavor

Instructions:

1. Slice sausage roll into ½-inch patties at indicated marks. (For less complicated slicing, area sausage in the freezer for 10-15 mins before slicing.)

2. Place patties in a chilly skillet. Cook over MEDIUM warmth for 14-16 mins, turning sausage often for even browning, or until the middle of sausage patty reaches 160°F and is no longer pink.

McDonald's McGriddle Breakfast Sandwich Servings

Servings: 5 servings

Nutrition: Carbohydrates: 6g/ Protein: 18g/ Fat: 31g

Ingredients:

For the pancake buns

- 3 eggs
- 4 tablespoons cream cheese
- 2 tablespoons grass-fed butter
- 1 teaspoon vanilla
- 1 1/2 cups almond flour
- 1 tablespoon Lankan to sugar
- 1 1/4 teaspoons baking soda
- 1/4 teaspoon salt
- 2 tablespoons Lankan to maple-flavored sugar-free syrup For the egg & meat portion
- 1 cooked egg
- 1 sausage patty
- 1 slice provolone cheese

Instructions:

1. In a big bowl, add all elements for the pancake buns and mix.

2. Add 2 tablespoons of pancake batter to the mini waffle maker and let prepare dinner for 2 mins.

3. Cook the egg and sausage as regular and upload it to the sandwich.

4. Enjoy sparkling or wrap in plastic wrap, seal in a freezer-secure bag after which freeze until ready to eat. Once prepared, eliminate from the plastic wrap and microwave for 30-40 seconds.

French Toast with Apple and Raisins

Ingredients:

- Raw egg 1 pcs
- Skimmed milk 1 cup
- Sweetener 1 CS
- Clove, ground 1 pinch (s)
- French toast bread 1 pcs (big ones)
- Apple without shell 1 pcs stings
- Seedless white raisins ¼ cups
- Light margarine 1 cs, melted
- Cinnamon powder 1 pinch (s)

Instructions:

1. Grease a medium refractory pan with spray oil and set aside.

Apart, beat the egg gently and add the milk, sweetener, and cloves, combining well. Add the bread cubes, apples, and raisins, blending lightly. Set aside until the bread absorbs all of the liquid.

2. In a bowl, integrate margarine and cinnamon. Spread the bread with the apple in the reserved form. Cover with cinnamon mixture. Bake in a reasonably preheated oven (180 ° C) for 30 minutes or till golden brown.

Meatloaf with Sweet Potato

Ingredients:

Meatloaf:

- 800 g of ground beef (duckling or rump)
- 1 envelope of onion cream
- 2 eggs
- 3 cloves garlic, minced
- 1 onion, finely chopped1/2 cup minced green smell salt to taste Filling:
- 2 chopped seedless tomatoes
- 1 chopped onion
- 1 large grated carrot Salt and pepper to taste catupiry (curd or grated mozzarella)

Other Ingredients:

- 12 to 15 bacon slices
- 5 sweet potatoes cut in 4 (pre-steamed)
- 3 thick sliced onions olive oil

Preparation:

Filling:

1. Mix tomatoes, onions, carrots, Salt, and pepper in a bowl.

Reserve.

Meatloaf:

2. In another bowl, mix all ingredients of the meatloaf properly.

3. With your hands, open the aggregate on the pinnacle of a plastic wrap or open plastic bag (this could make it easier to roll up).

4. Spread the filling.

5. Put the cheese of your choice (catupiry, curd, or mozzarella).

6. Close the roll, like a roll, and top with the bacon slices.

7. In a baking dish, unfold a drizzle of olive oil and make a layer with the onions in slices. Place the meatloaf over it.

8. On the sides, upload the remaining onions and candy potatoes.

9. Bake (at 220°C) for about 30 minutes till well browned.

Additional Information

Tips & Warnings Instead of sweet potatoes, use ordinary potatoes. The filling can be modified according to your creativity. Add black olives, palm hearts, or grated cabbage, for example. The mixture must be dehydrated so as not to drop water while ultimate and to bake the roll. Therefore, use tomatoes without the seed. If necessary, close the ends of the roll with barbecue sticks.

But take into account to take them out while serving. To accompany green salad and white rice. The onion cream and bacon already have enough Salt.

Be cautious while including more.

Cracker Barrel Meatloaf

Ingredients:

- 1 1/2 lb. ground chuck - 2 eggs
- 1 cup of crushed Ritz cracker
- 1/4 cup milk
- 1/2 cup finely chopped white onion
- Finely chopped blue peppers 1/4 cup
- 14.1 oz. canned tomato-can drain
- 1 tsp salt
- Black tea pepper 1/4 teaspoon
- Meatloaf glaze
- 1/2 cup ketchup
- 2 tablespoons brown sugar
- 1 tsp yellow mustard
- 1 tsp Worcester sauce

Instructions:

1. Meatloaf Glaze Preparation

2. Ketchup, brown sugar, mustard, and Worcestershire sauce are mixed in a small bowl.

3. Meatloaf Preparation

4. Preheat oven to 350 tiers F. For smooth removal, if wanted, line a baking sheet with parchment paper or aluminum foil.

5. Beat the eggs properly in a large bowl, then upload the crumbs of cracker, onion, inexperienced pepper, milk, salt, diced tomatoes drained, and pepper. Play well with each other.

6. Add red meat to the ground and blend properly. Shape the meatloaf aggregate into a loaf onto the prepared pan.

7. Bake and spread over the meatloaf for a half-hour. Bake for another 30 minutes or till 160 ° F is within the middle.

8. Let relaxation for 5-10 minutes, then slice and serve.

Nutrition

Calories: 253kcal | Carbohydrates: 12g | Protein: 14g | Fat: 16g | Saturated Fat: 6g | Cholesterol: 82mg | Sodium: 472mg | Potassium: 347mg | Fiber: 1g | Sugar: 7g | | Calcium: 51mg | Iron: 2mg

Senate bean soup with ham

Ingredients:

- 1 pound
- marine beans (or broad northern beans, dried, washed and drained)
- 1 bone of meaty ham (or 2 smoked hocks)
- 3 medium potatoes (cooked and mashed)
- 1 1/2 cups of onion (chopped)
- 1 1/2 cups of celery (chopped)
- 2 tablespoons of parsley (fresh, chopped)
- 2 large cloves garlic (minced) Salt to taste
- Black pepper to taste

Instructions:

1. Cover the beans with water and cook dinner for two minutes.

Remove from warmness, cover, and allow 1 to two hours to stand.

2. Place the colander on a bowl and pour the liquid from the beans.

Measure and upload sufficient water or unsalted vegetable soup to make 2 liters. Pour the liquid into the beans and upload the ham bone or ham hook, onions, celery, and garlic.

3. Bring to a boil the beans. Reduce warmth to a minimum, cowl the pan, and cook dinner for approximately 2 hours, or until very tender beans. Attach the mashed potatoes, carrots, celery, parsley, and garlic and cook for every other hour. Cut the bone or hocks from the ham and cut from the bones the beef. Cut the meat and placed it back in the soup. Season with Salt and pepper.

Tips

Bring the soup to a potluck or party. Transfer the cooked hot soup to a gradual cooker and placed it on low to serve.

Nutritional guidelines: Calories 274/ Fat 1 g/ Saturated fats 0 g/ Unsaturated fats 0 g/ Cholesterol 2 mg/ Sodium 109 mg/ Carbohydrates 52 g/ Dietary fiber 13 g/ Protein 15 g

Chick fil A sandwich

Ingredients:

- Marinade - 2 cups of water - 2 cube chicken bouillon - 1/4 teaspoon of seasoned salt
- Bread crumbs - 1 cup general purpose flour
- 1 1/2 cup finely ground salty cracker crumbs
- 2 teaspoon powdered sugar - 1/4 teaspoon paprika

Ingredients for sandwiches

- 4 hamburger buns - 8 dill pickles - 2 tablespoons butter
- You can use peanut oil vegetable oil for frying

Instructions:

1. Chicken marinade procedure

2. Add bloodless water to the bowl, upload 1/four teaspoon of seasoned salt and dissolve the bouillon cube in the mixture. Put bird breasts in water, mix, cowl, and refrigerate for 12 hours or the following day.

3. Chicken dough steps

4. Pour the hen marinade and discard it. It cannot be used again. In a small bowl, mix universal flour, crackers, powdered sugar, and paprika. Shuffle to combine.

5. Shake off extra marinade and sprinkle flour on the bird.

6. Place the beaten chook breasts on a twine rack and depart for a few minutes.

7. Cooking chicken

8. Heat the oil to 350 stages in a tempura pan or large pan. If you are the usage of a large pot, upload enough oil so that the oil is 4 inches deep.

9. Cook the fowl for 7-8 mins or till the chook turns brown and the internal temperature reaches 165 ° C. Drain the bird into a clean cord rack.

10. Collect sandwiches

11. Melt the butter and smooth with a burger roll.

12. Place one fowl sandwich on each bottom of the hamburger. Pickles of two dills, and top bread.

Nutrition: Calories: 781kcal | Carbohydrates: 69g | Protein: 35g | Fat: 40g | Saturated Fat: 10g | Cholesterol: 87mg | Sodium: 1956mg | Potassium: 667mg | Fiber: 4g | Sugar: 6g | Vitamin A: 508IU | Vitamin C: 3mg | Calcium: 149mg | Iron: 5mg

Fat Ronnie's Deep Fried Fresh Mushrooms

Ingredients:

- 2 cups of flour
- 1 1/2 teaspoon of Salt
- 1 teaspoon of ground pepper
- 1/2 teaspoon of baking soda
- 1 cup of buttermilk
- 8 ounces of fresh mushrooms (washed, dried, and stalks removed) Vegetable oil for frying

Instruction:

1. Preheat vegetable oil to 375 tiers.

2. Mix the flour, salt, pepper, and baking powder in a bowl. Put the buttermilk in a bowl.

3. Battering mushrooms

4. Shake out extra flour into the seasoned flour. Layer the buttermilk with the floured mushrooms.

5. Coat the buttermilk within the mushrooms, shake off excess buttermilk.

6. Return the mushrooms to the pro flour. Shake off buttermilk in abundance.

7. Cook mushrooms 1 to two minutes or golden brown until turning. Be sure to stir the mushrooms and cook dinner them on both sides.

8. Drain mushrooms in a bar pan on a twine rack.

Nutrition: 264kcal Carbohydrates: 35 g Protein: 6 g Fat: 10 g Saturated fat: 8 g Sodium: 626 mg Sodium: 252 mg Fiber: 1 g Sugar: 2 g Vitamin A: 65 IU Vitamin C: 0.8 mg Calcium: 67 mg Iron: 2.2 mg

Turkey Devonshire Sandwich like Armstrongs

Ingredients:

- cheese sauce
- 4 tablespoons of butter
- 4 tablespoons of flour
- 1 cup of chicken broth
- 1 cup whole milk
- 8 oz grated cheddar cheese I recommend a spicy cheddar, Tillamook
- 1/4 cup parmesan cheese cut into pieces sandwich 5 slices of bacon cooked
- 4 slices of Italian bread lightly toasted
- 4 slices of tomato
- 1/2 pound of turkey breast Paprika

Instructions:

Preheat the broiler.

Sauce instructions

1. Melt butter in a medium-sized saucepan and sprinkle with flour.

Cook over medium warmness the butter and flour aggregate for about a minute until the meal starts to odor nutty. Add 1 cup of broth of hen and 1 cup of milk and stir till thickened.

2. Add the sauce with Cheddar and Parmesan cheese, stir until the cheese melts. Remove the pan from the hot burner and stir once in a while because the sandwich is assembled to save your skin from growing on the pinnacle of the sauce.

Sandwich Assembly

Toast the bread.

3. Create a slice by installing a pie pan, a slice of toasted bread, top with turkey, and then tomato. Over the sandwich, ladle cheese sauce. Sprinkle on the pinnacle with a few paprikas.

4. Place the cheese sauce with slices of bacon crisscrossed. Broil until browning begins with cheese.

Nutrition: Calories: 1423kcal Carbohydrate: 43 g Protein: 74 g Fat: 106 g Saturated fat: 58 g Cholesterol: 300 mg Sodium: 2327 mg Potassium: 964 mg Fiber: 2 g Sugar: 21 g Vitamin A: 2592IU Vitamin C: 16 mg Calcium: 1129 mg Iron: 4 mg

Hooters hot wings

Ingredients:

- Cut 5 pounds of chicken wings in two, the drum and the side part 2 cups of whole wheat flour
- 1 cup of all-purpose flour
- 2 1/2 teaspoons of Salt
- 1 teaspoon of paprika
- 1/4 teaspoon of cayenne pepper

Instructions:

1. Layer flours, Salt, paprika, and cayenne pepper collectively and layer well in a massive blending bowl. Split the bird wings into the flappers and drumettes. Wash the chicken and drain it. Coat the bird in a mixture of flour; cool the chook wings for 90 minutes.

2. Split the fowl wings into the flappers and drumettes. Wash and drain chook.

3. Coat the bird in a combination of flour; cool the fowl wings for 90 mins.

4. When the chicken wings are prepared to fry, warm oil to 375 degrees. Place portions of fowl in hot oil, however do not crowd.

Fry the sides of the chook to a golden brown. Remove and drain from the oil. Place in a large bowl while all the wings were fried.

Remove the aggregate of warm sauce and blend properly. Place fowl portions on a serving platter, the usage of a fork or tongs.

Serve with lots of paper towels immediately.

California Pizza Kitchen Chicken Tequila Fettuccine

Ingredients:

- 1-2 pound dry spinach fettuccine (or 2 pounds fresh)
- 1/2 cup chopped coriander (2 tablespoons to garnish/finish)
- 2 tablespoons of chopped fresh garlic
- 2 tablespoons of chopped jalapeno pepper (seeds and veins can be removed if a milder flavor is desired)
- 3 tablespoons of unsalted butter (reserve tablespoons per saute)
- 1/2 cup chicken broth
- 2 tablespoons of tequila
- 2 tablespoons of freshly squeezed lime juice
- 3 tablespoons of soy sauce
- 1/2 pounds of chicken breast diced 3/4 inch
- 1/4 cup red onion thinly sliced
- 1 1/2 cup red pepper cut into thin slices
- 1/2 cup yellow pepper cut into thin slices
- 1/2 cup of green pepper cut into thin slices
- 1 1/2 cups of cream

Instructions:

1. Prepare speedy boiling salted water for pasta cooking; cook dinner till al dente, for dry pasta for 8 to 10 minutes, for sparkling for about three mins. Pasta may be cooked slightly in advance, rinsed and oiled after which "flashed" in boiling water or cooked to match with the sauce/topping finish.

2. Cook 1/3 cup cilantro, garlic, and jalapeno over medium warmness for four to 5 minutes in 2 tablespoons oil. Remove lime juice, tequila, and stock. Bring the combination to a boil and cook to a paste-like consistency till it is reduced; set aside.

3. Pour over the diced chook soy sauce; set apart for 5 mins.

Meanwhile, prepare dinner onion and peppers with the final butter over medium warmth, stirring on occasion. Toss and add reserved te q uila/lime paste and cream when the vegetables have wilted (become limp), add the chook and soy sauce.

4. Bring the sauce to a boil; cook gently till the hen is melted, and the sauce is thick (approximately 3 minutes).

Nutrition: Calories: 1077kcal Carbohydrates: 91 g Protein: 57 g Fat: 51 g Saturated fat: 28 g Sodium: 1057 mg Potassium: 1204 mg Fiber: 5 g Sugar: 5 g Vitamin A: 2600IU Vitamin C: 89.2 mg Calcium: 119 mg Iron: 3.5 mg

Chinese spare ribs

Ingredients:

- 1 tablespoon of hoisin sauce
- 1 teaspoon of toasted sesame oil
- 2 tablespoons of soy sauce
- 2 tablespoons of mirin or dry sherry
- 1/2 teaspoon of five-spice powder
- 2 tablespoons of chopped garlic
- 2 tablespoons of honey
- 2 tablespoons of ketchup
- 2 pounds of pork ribs

Instructions:

1. Combine Hoisin sauce, sesame oil, soy sauce, rice cooking vinegar, 5-spice powder, chopped garlic, butter, and ketchup in a medium-sized cup. Replace until the sauce is mixed. Pour over the ribs of red meat and marinate for at the very least 1 hour. If you may let them marinate a touch longer, these taste better.

Bake for 40 to 50 mins at 375.

Nutrition: Calories: 341kcal | Carbohydrates: 11g | Protein: 30g | Fat: 18g | Saturated fat: 3g | Cholesterol: 111mg | Sodium: 562mg | Potassium: 519mg | Fiber: 0g| Sugar: 9g | Vitamin A: 40IU | Vitamin C: 1.1mg | Calcium: 40mg | Iron: 1.6mg

California Pizza Kitchen Pumpkin Cheesecake

Ingredients:

- Graham Cracker Crust
- 1 1/2 cups of Graham Cracker Crumbs about 22 sheets 3 tablespoons of sugar
- 6 tablespoons of unsalted butter melted
- Cheesecake Filling
- 24 ounces of cream cheese
- 1 1/2 cups of dark brown sugar
- 1 tablespoon of all-purpose flour plus
- 2 teaspoons of all-purpose flour
- 1 1/2 teaspoon of ground cinnamon
- 1/8 teaspoon of ground cardamom
- 1/8 teaspoon of ground cloves
- 1/8 teaspoon of ground ginger
- 1/8 teaspoon of ground nutmeg
- 1 cup of sour cream plus
- 2 tablespoons of sour cream
- 3 eggs
- 2 teaspoons of vanilla extract
- 1 1/4 cups of canned pumpkin puree

Instructions:

To Make the Crust

1. In a meals processor equipped with the steel blade, area the graham cracker crumbs and procedure them until they have a uniformly first-class texture. Add the sugar and add the pulse.

2. The melted butter is progressively pumped into the feed tube while the machine is running and keeps processing until the aggregate paperwork a soft mass. Remove the combination from the processor and press it firmly into the base of a 9-inch springform pan to ensure that it's far lightly spread.

To Make the Cheesecake

3. Preheat the oven to 350 ° C.

4. Beat the cream cheese inside the blending bowl till it softens, sometimes stopping the mixer from scraping down the sides and bottom of the pan with a rubber spatula, the use of the flat beater attachment of your electric mixer.

5. Add the brown sugar and beat until the sugar is ultimately included, and the combination is creamy.

6. Mix the flour, cardamom, cinnamon, ginger, cloves, and nutmeg in a separate small bowl.

7. Whisk the aggregate of cream cheese and flour with a mixer till well combined. Stop now, after which to scrape the bowl's sides.

Stir one after the other within the sour cream and the eggs and wipe the pan after every addition.

8. Remove the pumpkin and vanilla and mix nicely.

9. Pour the filling into the organized springform pan's crust and place it for your oven's middle shelf. Bake for one hour. Test to peer if the cheesecake is ready to shake the pan gently to peer if the middle is the nearly firm-a sign of a casserole. (Alternatively, you may use a 180-diploma quick-read thermometer.) 10. Let it cool while the cheesecake is finished. Place overnight in the fridge before casting off the pan sides. Then reduce the cheesecake into thick slices, use a pointy knife. Tap here to see how to extract from the springform pan your cheesecake.

Nutrition: Calories: 357kcal Carbohydrate: 33 g Protein: 4 g Fat: 23 g Saturated fat: 13g Cholesterol: 97 mg Sodium: 220 mg Potassium: 171 mg Fiber: 0 g Sugar: 26 g Vitamin A: 3825IU Vitamin C: 0.9 mg Calcium: 95 mg Iron: 1.1

Homemade Copycat Olive Garden Zuppa Toscana

Ingredients:

- 1 pound of sweet or spicy Italian sausages
- 1 pound Russet potatoes, peeled, halved lengthways, then cut into 1/4 inch slices
- 1 cup of chopped onion
- 29 oz chicken broth 2 cans
- 1 liter of water
- 2 teaspoons of chopped garlic
- 1/4 cup Oscar Mayer Real Bacon Bits (1/2 box)
- salt and pepper
- 2 cups of chopped kale
- 1 cup of cream

Instructions:

Preheat the oven to 300 F. Place the sausages in a baking pan and roast until cooked through for approximately 30 mins. Drain and cut into slices on paper towels. Put the potatoes, onions, bird broth, water, and garlic in a pot and cook over medium heat till the potatoes are finished. Attach the sausage, bacon, salt, and pepper for another 10 minutes to taste and prepare dinner.

Turn the warmth down. If required, add kale, cream, and more tea. Cook and drink thoroughly.

Nutrition: Calories: 382kcal Carbohydrate: 15 g Protein: 12 g Fat: 30 g Saturated fat: 13g Cholesterol: 87 mg Sodium: 878 mg Potassium: 613 mg Fiber: 1 g Sugar: 1g Vitamin A: 2110IU Vitamin C: 33.6 mg Calcium: 78 mg Iron: 1.7 mg

SNACKS AND SIDE RECIPES

Potato skins loaded by TGI Friday

Servings: 4servings

Nutrition: Carbohydrates: 0g/ Protein: 4g/ Fat: 9g

Ingredients:

- 4 small russet potatoes - 1 tablespoon of olive oil
- 1 tablespoon of melted butter - 1/2 cup sharp cheddar cheese, shredded
- 1/4 cup mozzarella, shredded - 1/2 cup fried bacon, crumbled
- Salt and pepper - 1 cup sour cream - 1 chopped green onion

Instructions:

1. Preheat your oven to 425

2. Scrub the potatoes thoroughly, and permit them to dry

3. Pierce each potato 4-five time with a fork

4. Rub potatoes with olive oil and season lightly with salt and pepper to taste

5. Bake on a baking sheet covered with foil or parchment paper for 1 hour

6. Allow the potatoes to cool. When potatoes are cooled, set your oven to 375.

8. Cut each potato in half of lengthwise.

9. Using a spoon, lightly scoop out most (but now not all) of the white inner from each potato. You need to purpose to leave approximately 1/four inch in each skin. The relaxation of the scooped-out potato can be set aside and used for some other dish.

10. Melt the butter and brush the insides of the potato skins. Bake them hollow-side down for about 10 mins.

11. Remove the potatoes, brush the outside of the skins with butter, and gently flip them over (hollow-side up). Bake for another 15 mins, or till the skin receives crispy and the rims start to brown.

12. Sprinkle the cheese and bacon over the potato skins and return then to the oven for some mins till melted and bubbling.

13. Serve with sour cream and inexperienced onion!

Cracker Barrel's Biscuits

Servings: 10 biscuits

Nutrition: Carbohydrates: 47g/ Protein: 20g/ Fat: 22g

Ingredients:

- 2¼ cups Bisquick
- 2/3 cup buttermilk
- 1 teaspoon sugar
- 1 tablespoon butter, melted
- melted butter, for brushing

Instructions:

1. Preheat oven to 450°F.

2. Mix the Bis q uick, buttermilk and sugar together in a bowl.

3. Add the melted butter into the batter.

4. Stir till a smooth dough forms.

5. Turn out onto a well floured work surface.

6. Knead 20 times (this is a very forgiving dough), and don't be afraid to get extra flour into the dough.

7. Roll 1/2 thick, or thicker if you opt for towering biscuits.

8. Cut out into 2" rounds (or your preferred size).

9. Place close collectively on an ungreased baking sheet.

10. Brush tops with melted butter.

11. Bake for 8 to 10 minutes; I generally locate eight minutes is enough.

12. When you put off the biscuits from the oven, brush the tops with melted butter again.

Avocado Eggrolls from The Cheesecake Factory
Servings: 8 egg rolls

Nutrition: Carbohydrates: 27.7g/ Protein: 5.7g/ Fat: 18.4g

Ingredients:

- 1 cup vegetable oil
- 3 avocados, halved, peeled and seeded
- 1 Roma tomato, diced
- 1/4 cup diced red onion
- 2 tablespoons chopped fresh cilantro leaves
- Juice of 1 lime
- Kosher salt and freshly ground black pepper, to taste 8 egg roll wrappers
- 3/4 cup fresh cilantro leaves, loosely packed
- 1/3 cup sour cream
- 1 jalapeno, seeded and deveined, optional
- 2 tablespoons mayonnaise
- 1 clove garlic
- Juice of 1 lime
- Kosher salt and freshly ground black pepper, to taste

Instructions:

1. To make the cilantro dipping sauce, combine cilantro, sour cream, jalapeno, mayonnaise, garlic and lime juice in the bowl of a food processor; season with salt and pepper to taste. Set apart.

2. Heat vegetable oil in a big skillet or Dutch oven over medium excessive heat.

3. In a medium bowl, lightly mash avocados the use of a potato masher. Add tomato, pink onion, cilantro, lime juice, salt, and pepper, to taste, and lightly toss to combine.

4. Working one at a time, location avocado aggregate in the center of each wrapper. Bring the lowest edge of the wrapper tightly over the filling, folding within the sides. Continue rolling until the pinnacle of the wrapper is reached. Using your finger, rub the edges of the wrapper with water, pressing to seal. Repeat with remaining wrappers and avocado aggregate.

5. Working in batches, upload egg rolls to the Dutch oven and fry until lightly golden brown and crispy, approximately 2-three minutes. Transfer to a paper towel-covered plate.

6. Serve immediately with cilantro dipping sauce.

Easy Boiled Cabbage

Ingredients:

- Half cabbage
- 6 cloves of garlic
- ½ chili pepper
- 60 ml of extra virgin olive oil
- Salt and pepper

Preparation:

1. Wash and reduce the cabbage into portions, first in 1/2, after which every 1/2 into smaller pieces. Add a liter and a 1/2 of water in a casserole, a little salt, and a bay leaf. When the water boils, upload the cabbage. Cook for 8 mins after which drain and reserve.

2. Cut the garlic cloves into large pieces and the chili pepper, add virgin olive oil to a nonstick skillet.

3. Sauté the garlic for 2 or three minutes so that they brown if burned. Then remove the garlic from the pan; however, go away the chili. Now add the well-drained cabbage and simmer for 7-10 mins, upload Salt and pepper and allow stand a few minutes before serving.

Frijoles Negros (Cuban Black Beans)

Ingredients:

- 450 grams of black beans
- 10 cups of Water (2400 milliliters)
- 6 tablespoons olive oil - 1 unit large onion
- 5 cloves of garlic - ¼ tablespoon oregano dessert
- 1 bay leaf
- ¼ tablespoon ground cumin dessert
- 1 pinch of Salt
- 1 pinch of pepper
- 1 tablespoon vinegar
- 1 tablespoon dry wine
- 1 tablespoon of sugar

Preparation:

1. 1 unit sizeable green chili pepper Steps to follow to make this recipe:

2. To begin with our recipe for Cuban beans, the primary thing we're going to do is to wash the seeds correctly and soak them with water and a bay leaf. Ideally, leave them overnight so that they inflate, and you could cook dinner them better.

3. The subsequent day, take a pot with enough capacity, pour the beans in it with the water and the bay leaf and cook dinner them for approximately forty-five minutes until they're gentle.

4. When they are equipped, drain them and prepare the black bean stir fry. To do this, take a deep pan and warmth the olive oil. Once hot, add the finely chopped onion and chili, or overwhelmed if desired, and overwhelmed garlic. Remove it with a timber spoon and fry it. Of the already smooth beans, reserve a cup for later; the rest add it to the frypan, with the blade included. Remove everything, upload salt and pepper to taste, oregano, cumin, and sugar and simmer for a couple of minutes. Do not stop stirring to prevent black beans from sticking and burning.

5. Then, mash the beans you reserved in the cup, add them to the rest and simmer them for half of an hour and with the pan covered. After the time, add the dry wine and the vinegar, stir it properly and let it rest with the fire for a minimum of 10 minutes. When they may be prepared to feature tablespoons of olive oil, integrate it and serve the black beans to the Cuban accompanied with the aid of white rice.

Nutrition: Calories: 172kcal Carbohydrates: 18 g Protein: 6 g Fat: 9 g Saturated fat: 5 g Sodium: 294 mg Potassium: 369 mg Fiber: 7 g Sugar: 1 g Vitamin A: 111IU Vitamin C: 9 mg Calcium: 23 mg Iron: 1 mg

Carrot Pudding

Ingredients:

- 3 cups grated carrots
- one cup of water
- two cardamom seeds
- two teaspoons vanilla
- 1/4 cup evaporated milk
- 1/2 cup of condensed milk
- 1/4 cup cashews (cashews), cut, if desired

Instructions:

1. In a 2-quart pot over low warmness, blend the water, cardamom seeds and vanilla, permit it to boil. When the water has boiled, add the carrots, stir and cover. Cook with the pot blanketed for 10 minutes.

2. After 10 minutes, find the pot and upload evaporated milk and condensed milk. Cook without a lid, occasionally stirring till the maximum of the liquid is absorbed, which takes approximately 20 minutes.

3. Remove from warmness and upload chopped cashews, if desired. Take a spoon and get prepared to enjoy a delicious dessert!

Nutrition: Calories: 296kcal Carbohydrate: 40 g Protein: 4 g Fat: 13 g Saturated fat: 8 g Cholesterol: 112 mg Sodium: 211 mg Potassium: 424 mg Fiber: 3 g Sugar: 30 g Vitamin A: 19420IU Vitamin C: 6.7 mg Calcium: 64 mg Iron: 1 mg 84.

Copycat Cracker barrel sprouts and kale salad

Ingredients:

- 1 bunch of kale
- 1 pound of Brussels sprouts
- 16 ounces. Bag Craisins
- 8 ounces. chopped pecans
- Maple Vinaigrette
- 1/2 c. olive oil
- 1/4 c. Apple Cider Vinegar
- 4 Tbs. maple syrup
- 1 teaspoon. dry mustard

Instructions:

1. Sprinkle or thinly slice the kale and Brussel and installed a salad bowl.

2. Toast pecans for 60-ninety seconds in a skillet over high heat.

3. Bowl with pecans and craisins.

4. Mix well all the elements of the vinaigrette.

5. Pour over salad vinaigrette and mix to cowl evenly. Let at least four hours or overnight stay within the fridge.

Nutrition: Calories: 357kcal Carbohydrates: 42 g Protein: 5 g Fat: 21 g Saturated fat: 12g Sodium: 334 mg Potassium: 503 mg Fiber: 3 g Sugar: 31 g Vitamin A: 4598IU Vitamin C: 97 mg Calcium: 116 mg Iron: 2 mg

Garlic Green Beans

Ingredients:

- 800 g of fresh green beans
- 2 cloves of garlic
- 1 tablet of vegetable broth
- 1 teaspoon chopped thyme
- 1 lemon
- 2 tablespoons olive oil salt

Preparation:

1. Cut the ends of the beans, get rid of the strands, and chop them.

Peel and crush the garlic cloves collectively with the thyme in a mortar. Put the oil in a pan and sauté the beans three or four minutes, upload the mashed garlic, and saute 3 extra mins over low heat without letting the garlic burn.

2. Add water just to cover, pour the crumbled broth, and salt to flavor. Cook till the beans are tender (approximately 15-20 minutes), drain them, and water them with the lemon juice.

Nutrition: Calories: 175kcal Carbohydrates: 17 g Protein: 4 g Fat: 12 g Saturated fat: 7g Cholesterol: 30 mg Sodium: 114 mg Potassium: 479 mg Fiber: 6 g Sugar: 7g Vitamin A: 1915IU Vitamin C: 29 mg Calcium: 89 mg Iron: 2 mg

Oven Roasted Brussel Sprouts

Ingredients:

- 500 grams of Brussels sprouts
- 3 tablespoons olive oil
- 2 tablespoons balsamic vinegar of Modena
- 2 tablespoons honey (or agave syrup or another sugar-free substitute) Salt to taste
- Ground black pepper to taste Steps to observe to make this recipe:

Preparation:

1. Wash the cabbages and put off the top layers when necessary.

We split them in half. Place the cabbage in a bowl and add the olive oil. We blend well.

2. Then, add the vinegar, honey, or syrup and season to flavor. We blend well.

3. Place the mixture on a baking sheet lined with vegetable paper with the internal of the cabbages dealing with up, and prepare dinner the Brussels sprouts inside the oven and warm at 200°C at half-height approximately 20 minutes till golden brown and tender.

4. You will see how wealthy the roasted Brussels sprouts are left with that bittersweet mixture and the golden-brown of the oven.

I can't think about a better manner to enjoy this vegetable.

Really, superior!

Nutrition: Calories: 265kcal Carbohydrates: 22 g Protein: 8 g Fat: 19 g Saturated fat: 3g Sodium: 639 mg Potassium: 911 mg Fiber: 9 g Sugar: 6 g Vitamin A: 1710IU Vitamin C: 194 mg Vitamin C: 100 mg Iron: 3 mg

Baked beans with smoked sausage

Ingredients:

- 2 slices of bacon, chopped into 1/2 inch pieces 1 sweet onion, chopped
- 2 cloves of garlic, finely chopped
- 1/2 pound smoked sausage, sliced, I use Kielbasa 3 (16 oz.) Cans of pork and beans
- 1/2 cup of ketchup
- 1/3 cup light brown sugar
- 1/4 cup molasses
- 2 tablespoons of apple cider vinegar
- 2 tablespoons of yellow mustard
- 1/4 to 1/2 teaspoon of hot sauce, use TABASCO

Instructions:

1. Heat the oven as much as 350 degrees.

2. Cook bacon till crispy in a Dutch oven. With a slotted spoon, do away with and put on a towel-covered sheet of paper.

3. Add the onion and prepare dinner until soft to the bacon drippings. Add the garlic and smoked sausage and cook until browned with the sausage.

4. Cut the rest of the ingredients. Bring it to low heat. Place the exposed Dutch oven in the oven and prepare dinner until thick for 45 to 55 minutes.

5. Calories of nutrition: 368kcal

Savory Mashed Purple Potatoes

Ingredients:

- 1 green apple - 4 violet potatoes - ½ onion - 1 tablespoon butter
- ½ cup of milk - Salt

Direction:

1. Wash the potatoes properly and vicinity them in a pot.

2. Cover with water and a pinch of salt.

3. Let cook over slight heat until smooth.

4. Chop the onion finely.

5. Heat a pan with the butter.

6. When it melts, upload the onion.

7. Saute for 5 mins over low heat.

8. Wash and peel the apple, doing away with the coronary heart and seeds.

9. Cut it into small pieces.

10. Add to the onion, sautéing for 3 more minutes.

11. Add the milk and raise the warmth.

12. When the boil breaks, decrease the heat and cook dinner for two mins.

13. Remove.

14. Place the preparation within the blender.

15. Crush to homogenize.

16. Peel the potatoes and overwhelm them with pureed raisins.

Season to taste.

17. Mix the mashed potatoes with the apple preparation.

18. Beat with the rods until you get a smooth and creamy puree.

Serve the mashed potatoes and violet apples boiling.

Nutrition: Calories: 195kcal Carbohydrates: 26 g Protein: 3 g Fat: 8 g Saturated fat: 5 g Cholesterol: 28 mg Sodium: 435 mg Potassium: 646 mg Fiber: 3 g Sugar: 1 g Vitamin A: 310IU Vitamin C: 29.8 mg Calcium: 27 mg Iron: 1.2 mg

Fried Zucchini

Ingredients:

- 2 large zucchini
- 2 eggs
- 1 cup of flour
- Olive oil
- Salt

Preparation:

1. We wash the zucchini well and reduce them into skinny slices, about 4 millimeters thick. When we've got them to reduce into sheets, the method is as follows:

2. With the new olive oil, first, we put each slice of zucchini in beaten egg, then in flour, and subsequently in egg again. And so we skip it to the pan.

3. If we fry with the hot oil, the zucchini slices may be crispy at the outdoor and soft at the inside: delicious!

4. Finally, as we take out the zucchini, we placed them on a plate with a paper serviette so that it absorbs the oil properly.

5. To eat!

Nutrition: Calories: 328kcal | Carbohydrates: 18g | Protein: 12g | Fat: 22g | Saturated Fat: 11g | Cholesterol: 301mg | Sodium: 340mg | Potassium: 312mg | Fiber: 1g | Sugar: 3g | Vitamin A: 570IU | Vitamin C: 11.7mg | Calcium: 94mg | Iron: 2.8mg

Bloomin 'Onion and Chili Sauce from Outback

Servings: 4 servings

Nutrition: Carbohydrates: 125g/ Protein: 15g/ Fat: 1g

Ingredients:

- ½ cup mayonnaise
- 2 table spoons prepared horseradish
- 2 teaspoon sketchup
- ¼ teaspoon paprika
- ¼ teaspoonsalt
- ⅛ teaspoon garlic powder
- ⅛ teaspoondried oregano
- Dash ground black pepper
- Dash cayenne pepper

Instructions:

1. In a small bowl, stir together all the ingredients till absolutely

combined.

2. Serve right now or cover and refrigerate until geared up to serve.

The leftover dipping sauce can be stored inside the refrigerator, covered, for up to one week.

Applebee spinach and artichoke sauce
Servings: 10 servings

Nutrition: Carbohydrates: 9g/ Protein: 13g/ Fat: 30g

Ingredients:

- 16 oz. roasted garlic alfredo sauce
- 8 ounces cream cheese, at room temperature
- ½ cup Parmesan cheese, shredded
- ½ cup Romano cheese, shredded
- 2 cups low-moisture whole milk mozzarella cheese, shredded 28 oz. artichoke hearts, drained/rinsed/chopped 16 oz. fresh spinach, steamed (can sub with 10 oz. frozen spinach)
- ½ cup milk, optional, use if you want the dip to be a little less
- thick

Instructions:

1. Add the alfredo sauce to a huge saucepan over medium heat.

2. Cut the cream cheese into cubes and blend it into the alfredo sauce till well-combined and creamy. Use a fork to whisk any lumps out.

3. Add the Parmesan, Romano, and Mozzarella cheeses and stir until properly-blended.

4. Stir within the artichoke hearts, then add the spinach. Stir until nicely combined

5. If the dip is thicker than desired, upload up to a ½ cup of milk and stir until blended and heated through.

6. Serve with tortilla chips, pita chips, fresh bread, and/or vegetables.

7. Store within the refrigerator for as much as 4 days.

Copycat Mozzarella Sticks by TGI Fridays

Servings: 4 servings

Nutrition: Carbohydrates: 77g/ Protein: 38g/ Fat: 30g

Ingredients:

- 1 pound mozzarella cheese
- 1 cup flour
- 1/4 cup cornstarch
- 2 cups Italian seasoned breadcrumbs
- 1 cup milk
- vegetable oil for frying

Instructions:

1. Cut cheese sticks into long slices approximately 3/8 inch thick.

Blend the flour and cornstarch collectively in a bowl. Place cheese plank into the flour, then dip into a bowl of whole milk, after which dip the cheese stick into the breadcrumbs.

2. Shake off excess breadcrumbs and place mozzarella stick on a card rack. Discard the flour. Repeat until all cheese sticks have been dipped once.

3. When all of the cheese sticks have been dipped once vicinity back into milk, then into bread crumbs for the second one time, and shake off the bread crumbs. Dip all cheese sticks into bread crumbs for the second time.

4. Preheat vegetable oil to 350 for frying. Drop cheese sticks into the warm oil and fry until golden brown. This has to take no longer than 1 minute. Remove cheese sticks from oil and location on a cord rack to cool. Serve with your favorite marinara sauce.

Pickled Deep Pickles of the Texas Roadhouse

Servings: 3 -4 yields

Nutrition: Carbohydrates: 10g/ Protein: 1g/ Fat: 14g

Ingredients:

- 3 cups dill pickle sliced
- 1 cup all-purpose flour
- 1 teaspoon Cajun seasoning
- 1/2 teaspoon dried oregano
- 1/2 teaspoon dried basil
- 1/4 teaspoon cayenne pepper
- 1 teaspoon salt
- 1/4 cup mayonnaise
- 1 tablespoon horseradish
- 1 tablespoon ketchup
- 1/4 teaspoon Cajun seasoning

Instructions:

1. In a small mixing bowl, mix the flour, Cajun seasoning, dried oregano, dried basil, cayenne pepper and salt.

2. Drain the pickles and then dried them on paper towels for approximately 20 minutes. So they would be ready for dredging.

3. Coat the pickles with the seasoned flour.

4. As you are making them placed the battered pickles on either an air fryer basket or tray (both have been sprayed with olive oil, so they don't stick)

5. Now, here is the secret, you MUST spray them all the batter with olive oil spray. So they grow to be crispy.

6. Set inside the air fryer oven or basket, and set the temperature to 400 tiers F, for 7 minutes, after 5 minutes, turn and air fry for any other 7 minutes (air fryer setting)

7. Meanwhile, in a small mixing bowl, mix the components for the dipping sauce collectively.

8. Plate, serve, and enjoy!

The famous Olive Garden breadsticks

Servings: 12 breadsticks

Nutrition: Carbohydrates: 27.5g/ Protein: 3.8g/ Fat: 4.7g

Ingredients:

- 1 cup plus 2 tablespoons warm water
- 1 1/2 teaspoons instant yeast
- 2 tablespoons granulated sugar
- 3 tablespoons unsalted butter, melted
- 1 3/4 teaspoons salt
- 16 ounces (about 3 1/3 to 3 1/2 cups) bread flour 2 tablespoons unsalted butter, melted
- 1/2 teaspoon kosher salt
- 1/4 teaspoon garlic powder

Instructions:

1. In the bowl of a standing mixer, combine the water, yeast, sugar, and butter. Add within the salt. Attach the dough hook to the mixer and start to upload the flour on low pace regularly.

Increase the velocity to medium and knead the dough for about 7 minutes, or until it is clean and elastic.

2. Remove the dough to a lightly oiled bowl and cowl with plastic wrap. Let relaxation in a warm region until doubled in size, approximately 1 half of hours.

3. Divide the dough into 12 (2 ounce) portions. Roll every piece of dough into a 7-inch log. Place the dough logs on nonstick baking mat or parchment-coated baking sheets, cowl, and let rise until doubled in size, about 1 hour.

4. Preheat the oven to 400°F. Bake for approximately 12 minutes, or till golden brown. Remove from oven and without delay brush with melted butter: Combine the salt and garlic powder and sprinkle evenly over breadsticks. Serve warm.

Copycat Krispy Kreme Donuts Glazed

Ingredient:

Donuts

- 2 1/4 teaspoons active dry yeast
- 1/2 cup warm water, 110 degrees
- 1/4 cup granulated sugar, divided
- 1/4 cup evaporated milk, heated to 110 degrees 1/2 teaspoon salt
- 1/4 cup shortening, at room temperature
- 1 large egg
- 1 egg yolk
- 1/2 teaspoon vanilla extract
- 2 1/2 cups all-purpose flour, then more as needed 3-4 cups of shortening, for frying

Glaze

- 2 tablespoons unsalted butter, melted
- 1 1/3 cups of powdered sugar
- 1 pinch of salt
- 2 teaspoons evaporated milk
- 1/2 teaspoon vanilla extract
- 3 - 4 teaspoons hot water

Direction:

1. In the bowl of an electric powered mixer, blend the yeast, warm water, and 1/2 teaspoon of sugar. Let stand 5 to 10 minutes.

2. Add the evaporated milk, the remaining granulated sugar (three tablespoons + 2 1/2 teaspoons), salt, 1/four cup butter, egg, egg yolk, and vanilla.

3. Add half the flour and modify the blender with the whisk and blend until smooth.

4. Change the blender to the hook attachment, slowly add the ultimate flour and knead at low speed till it's miles clean and elastic for about four to five minutes, adding extra flour as needed (I best brought about 2 tablespoons more.

5. You ought to no longer want a great deal more; you want the dough should be barely sticky and sticky, but ought to now not adhere to the top of the smooth finger). Transfer the mixture to a lightly greased bowl.

6. Knock the dough down and roll in a uniform layer on a floured floor with a thickness of less than half an inch. Donut-shaped cut with a donut cutter or two ound cutters (one massive and one small for holes). Cover and permit upward thrust till doubled, approximately 30 to 40 mins.

7. Reduce warmth in a Dutch reliable iron oven to 360 degrees (do no longer move away from oil during preheating and do not allow it to exceed 375 degrees, remove from warmness and decrease warmness as necessary).

8. Meanwhile, put together the glaze by way of mixing all of the glaze substances in a shallow dish (do not add too much water, you'll dip warm donuts within the enamel so that you don't need it to be liquid, pretty thick is good).

9. Carefully switch the donuts to the oil (it may fry three at a time) and fry until golden brown on the bottom, then use a timber stick, flip to the opposite aspect and cook the different facet until golden brown.

10. Transfer to a cord rack and let it cool for 1 to 2 minutes, then immerse the upper half inside the enamel while it is nonetheless warm and go back to the twine rack and permit the teeth to set at room temperature. Better served heat. Once cold, reheat within the microwave for five to ten seconds if preferred.

Roasted Pumpkin Seeds

Ingredients:

- 1 pumpkin
- Olive oil
- Salt
- Spices to taste (salt and pepper, paprika, cinnamon and sugar, curry, etc.)

Instructions:

1. We preheat the oven to 200 ° C (400 ° F)

2. Remove the pumpkin seeds

3. We get rid of the pulp from the seeds and wash them in cold water in a pot; we can boil the seeds, use 2 cups of water for every half cup of seeds

4. Add a teaspoon of salt for each cup of water and allow them to simmer for 10 minutes

5. We remove the water and dry

6. On a baking sheet, we put olive oil

7. We region the seeds on the pinnacle of the oil and season them to our liking

8. Bake for 25 to 40 minutes (till golden brown and crispy) I devour them as a whole - even though there are individuals who opt for to most effectively consume the small seed inside.

Nutrition: Calories: 72kcal Carbohydrates: 1 g Protein: 3 g Fat: 6 g Saturated fat: 1 g Sodium: 255 mg Potassium: 86 mg Fiber: 0 g Sugar: 0 g Vitamin A: 45IU Vitamin C: 0.2 mg Calcium: 5 mg Iron: 0.9 mg

Homemade Spicy Beef Jerky

Ingredients:

- 1 kg of roulades from a butcher or another lean beef, 4-5mm thick slices
- 100 ml soy sauce
- 150 ml organic apple cider vinegar
- 1 tbsp Sambal Oelek
- Salt pepper
- 1 pinch of stevia

Preparation:

1. Mix the elements for the marinade thoroughly.

2. Remove any fat from the beef and reduce it into the preferred portions.

3. Put the beef and marinade alternately in a meal bag.

4. If possible, squeeze the air out of the bag and seal it.

5. Leave to marinate within the fridge for twelve to 24 hours.

6. Drain, dab very well with kitchen paper.

7. Allow drying on a grid at around 50 degrees within the oven (go away the air and a small hole open) or within the digital dehydrator for approximately 8-10 hours.

Nutritional information:

Serving: 1 total | Calories: 860 kcal | Carbohydrates: 95 g | Protein: 48 g | Fat: 32 g

Caviar Deviled Eggs

The recipe for stuffed eggs with Caviar is one of the most natural methods that can be made, but also one of the richest. Who has not eaten them stuffed with tuna at any time? Well, in this case, we will prepare them with a sturgeon roe. The truth today, I do not know anyone who does not like, despite the simplicity of the recipe.

Ingredients:

- 4 eggs
- 2 tablespoons fresh cream
- 1/2 teaspoon paprika
- A pinch of salt
- 30 g of Caviar
- 1 sprig of fresh dill

Preparation:

1. Boil the eggs. Fill a saucepan with water, introduce the eggs, and placed them inside the stove. When it starts off evolved to boil, count 5 mins, and do away with from heat.

2. Cool them with water, and then cast off them carefully, to maintain the brilliant look of the egg.

3. Take a knife and reduce the eggs in half. With a spoon, get rid of the yolk from the inside, taking care now not to break the white part. Place all of the bears in a separate container.

4. To the yolks, add the sparkling cream and paprika. Mix well until a thin clean cream is made.

5. On a plate, place the halves of the eggs. Fill the interior with the aggregate you have created with the yolks. Cover with the sturgeon eggs which you have chosen on the pinnacle of the combination.

6. To decorate, sprinkle a few paprikas to provide it a hint of color.

Then put some dill leaves on the combination and after the caviar.

Nutrition: Calories: 106kcal Carbohydrate: 3 g Protein: 7 g Fat: 6 g Saturated fat: 2 g Cholesterol: 215 mg Sodium: 301 mg Potassium: 80 mg Fiber: 0 g Sugar: 1 g Vitamin A: 335IU Calcium: 39 mg Iron: 1.2 mg

APPETIZERS

Lasagna with Feta and Black Olives

Lasagna with Greek flavors, very easy to hop very quickly for the sun's return! I flavored it with a combination of Greek herbs returned from our summer holidays. It contains oregano, thyme, red pepper, basil, mint, and so on.

Ingredients:

- 8 lasagna sheets
- 600 gr of diced tomatoes
- Dried basil and oregano
- Salt and black pepper
- 1 sugar
- +/- 300 ml of béchamel
- 1 jar of pitted kalamata black olives
- +/- 150 gr of block feta
- A little grated cheese to brown
- A mixture of dried Greek herbs Olive oil

Preparation:

1. Heat a touch olive oil in a saucepan or frying pan. Add the diced tomatoes, sugar, dried basil and oregano, salt and pepper (dose in step with your taste). Let simmer for at least 1/2 hour. Prepare your béchamel as you commonly do. Drain the olives and dice the feta.

2. Spread a little tomato and béchamel sauce within the bottom of a gratin dish, location 2 sheets of lasagna, tomato sauce, béchamel, black olives, and diced feta. Continue identically till all the ingredients are used up. Finish with béchamel, sprinkle with grated cheese and sprinkle with Greek herbs.

3. Finally, bake at 180 ° C for 30 to 40 minutes and serve immediately.

Fried keto cheese with mushrooms

Ingredients:

- 300 g mushrooms
- 300 g halloumi cheese
- 75 g butter 10 green olives
- salt and ground black pepper
- 125 ml (125 g) mayonnaise (optional)

Instructions:

Rinse and trim the mushrooms and chop or slice them.

1. Heat the right quantity of butter in a pan in which they match and halloumi cheese and mushrooms.

2. Fry the mushrooms over medium heat for 3-5 minutes till golden brown. Salpimentarlos.

3. If vital, add extra butter and fry the halloumi cheese for a few minutes on every side. Stir the mushrooms occasionally.

4. Lower the warmness towards the end. Serve with olives.

Hooter's Buffalo Wings

Ingredients:

- 2 kilos of chicken wings separated in wing and thigh, defrosted, and well dried.
- 2 cups of regular flour
- 1 teaspoon of garlic powder
- 1 teaspoon of chili pepper
- 1 teaspoon of paprika or paprika
- 1 teaspoon of salt
- ½ teaspoon of ground black pepper
- Half bar of melted butter
- 2 cups of sauce, can be spicy wings, sold in supermarkets, it can be bbq sauce, you can mix both sauces to make the Daytona style, you can shacer your own mixture of sauces, I like to mix the Frank's Red Hot Wings sauce (they sell it in the Mexican commercial) with the sauce Kraft brand BBQ in equal parts. The important thing is to add the melted butter to give it the final touch.
- 1 liter of vegetable oil for frying

Preparation:

1. It is very critical that the wings are dry and wholly thawed, skip them on a towel to cast off all of the moisture. Mix the flour, salt, paprika, piquin chili, garlic, and pepper and breach the wings very well, allow them relaxation for at least an hour within the refrigerator and then re-pan them. If you want them without breading, do the same procedure; however, without flour, and it is not essential to refrigerate them before frying them, which ought to be cooked longer so that the skin will become golden brown.

2. Heat the oil in a deep and massive pan or a deep fryer and cook dinner the wings on each side until they are brown, however, without burning.

3. Remove the wings from the oil and dry them with paper to soak up the fat, when you're going to serve them, soak them within the sauce mixture. Serve with celery and ranch dressing or blue cheese.

Nutrition: Calories: 666kcal | Carbohydrates: 44g | Protein: 44g | Fats: 33g | Saturated Fat: 9g | Cholesterol: 157mg | Sodium: 1119mg | Potassium: 493mg | Fiber: 4g | Sugar: 0g | Vitamin A: 500 IU | Vitamin C: 1.4 mg | Calcium: 41mg | Iron: 4.4 mg

Veggie Patch Pizza

Ingredients:

- 300 gr. whole wheat flour
- Mozzarella cheese
- 1 envelope baker's baking powder
- 200 ml of warm water
- 2 tablespoons oil
- 1 teaspoon salt
- Tomato
- Bonduelle beet
- Bonduelle Piquillo
- Pepper black olives

Instructions:

1. Preheat oven to 350 ranges.

2. Spray with non-stick spray a vast cookie sheet. Roll out the cookie sheet with crescent rolls. Unroll the dough quickly, don't divide it into triangles. Press down flat on the indentations. Bake until golden brown for approximately 12-15 minutes. Until continuing, permit the cooked dough to chill.

3. Combine cream cheese, mayonnaise, dry ranch dressing blend, and dehydrated onion in a bowl in a medium-sized dish. Spread the combination of cream cheese over the cooked roll dough.

Finish with greens that uniformly scatter veggies over the pizza.

Cut proper away, even supposing you're no longer going always to do this. When you wait too long to reduce this, the dough may be pulled off through the cream cheese layer. You can make your Veggie Patch Pizza a day beforehand of time, but be sure to reduce it before you cowl it to save the Veggie Patch Pizza.

Easy Copycat Monterey's Little Mexico Queso

Ingredients:

- 1/2 cup of chopped yellow onion
- 1/2 cup of finely chopped celery
- 2 large green peppers such as Anaheim or Hatch, finely diced 2 tablespoons of butter
- 1 pound of American cheese
- 1/3 cup milk

Instructions:

1. The real mystery of flavored cheese is to fry vegetables till they're almost wholly cooked when you begin adding a little crunch in your American cheese.

2. Place the chopped onion, thinly sliced celery and diced pepper in a casserole over medium warmness, upload tablespoons of oil, and cook until the onion is transparent. Put in a medium bowl, American cheese, sautéed onions, and milk. Heat until low or medium warmness melts the cheese.

Nutrition: Calories: 226kcal Carbohydrates: 4 g Protein: 9 g Fat: 18 g Saturated fat: 10g Sodium: 57 mg Sodium: 874 mg Potassium: 169 mg Fiber: 0 g Sugar: 2 g Vitamin A: 730IU Vitamin C: 30.1 mg Calcium: 545 mg Iron: 0.5 mg

Olive Garden Fried Mozzarella

Ingredients:

- Sixteen ounces mozzarella cheese
- 2 eggs beaten 1/4 cup water
- 1 1/2 cups Italian breadcrumbs
- 1/2 teaspoons garlic salt
- 1 teaspoon Italian condiments
- 2/3 cup flour
- 1/3 cup cornstarch

Directions:

1. Cut it into thick slices at the same time as your cheese is in a brick and reduce it throughout to form triangles. Beat the water in the eggs and set apart. Blend collectively and set aside the breadcrumbs, garlic salt, and Italian spices. Mix and hold the cornstarch with the flour.

2. Heat 360 levels of vegetable oil.

3. Dip the cheese inside the flour and cornstarch combination, then cowl with the breadcrumbs within the beaten egg.

4. Place the cheese carefully in hot oil and fry till golden brown, so be patient. When golden brown, extract and drink from the new oil. Eat and revel in with your favorite sauce of Italian spaghetti.

Nutrition: Calories: 661kcal Carbohydrate: 59 g Protein: 36 g Fat: 30g Saturated fat: 16g Cholesterol: 171 mg Sodium: 1636 mg Potassium: 242 mg Fiber: 3 g Sugar: 3 g Vitamin A: 970IU Vitamin C: 1.2 mg Calcium: 678 mg Iron: 4.3mg

Shrimp nachos with avocado and tomato salsa

Ingredients:

- SALSA
- 2 ripe Hass avocados, diced ¼ inch
- 1 large ripened tomato, free of stems and seeds, cut into ¼-inch dice
- 2 tablespoons fresh lime juice
- 1 tablespoon finely chopped fresh coriander leaves 1 garlic clove, minced or garlic press
- ½ teaspoon ground cumin
- Kosher Salt
- Freshly ground black pepper
- 1 ear of sweet corn, peeled
- Extra virgin olive oil
- ½ teaspoon ground cumin
- ¼ teaspoons chipotle chili powder
- 20 jumbo shrimps (count of 21/30), shelled and deveined, without the tail
- 170 grams tortilla chips
- 225 grams of coarsely grated sharp cheddar cheese 4 green onions (white and pale green parts only), thinly sliced, green and white parts separated
- 1 small jalapeño pepper, seeded, finely chopped 1 tablespoon chopped fresh coriander

Instructions:

1. Combine the components for the salsa sauce. Season with ½ tsp.

Salt and ¼ tsp. Of pepper.

2. Prepare the grill for direct cooking over medium warmness (350 to 450 ° F) and preheat the perforated grill for 10 mins.

3. Lightly brush the corn with oil, then grill directly on the cooking grids over medium warmth, with the lid closed and turning it if necessary, till it is browned in places and tender, eight to 12 mins. Leave to cool, then cut the grains from the cob.

4. Mix the cumin, the chili powder, ½ tsp. Salt and ¼ tsp. Of pepper. Brush the shrimp with oil, then sprinkle the spice aggregate lightly. Divide the shrimp in a single layer on the baking sheet and grill over medium direct heat, with the lid closed and turning once till they're firm to the touch and opaque inside the center, 2 to 4 minutes. With protecting barbeque gloves, do away with the baking sheet and the shrimp from the warmth and transfer the shrimp to a piece surface. Cut every shrimp in 1/2 crosswise, crosswise.

5. Prepare the grill for oblique cooking over medium warmness (350 to 450 ° F).

6. Spread the tortilla chips on the bottom of a 12-inch solid iron skillet. Scatter cheese calmly over potato chips, then corn, the white part of green onions, and jalapeño pepper. Cook over indirect medium warmth, with the barbecue lid, closed, for 8 to 10 minutes, till the cheese has melted. During the final 2 mins of cooking, upload the shrimp on the nachos. Remove from warmth and garnish with the inexperienced a part of the green onions and the coriander. Serve warm with salsa.

Mimosa eggs with truffle

Ingredients:

- 6 Eggs
- 1/2 cup Mayonnaise
- 2 c. tablespoons Chives finely chopped
- 1-2 tsp. tablespoon truffle oil of excellent quality 2-3 slices crispy bacon, crumbled
- Salt and pepper
- Pastry bag or Ziploc bag

Instructions:

Boil the eggs for approximately 8 minutes. Let cool and peel the shell. Cut in 1/2 lengthwise, cast off the yolk with a small spoon, and place in a bowl with mayonnaise, truffle oil, salt, pepper, and half of the chives. Mash the mixture with a fork or use a small blender. Put all of the mixtures in a piping bag or a Ziploc bag. Arrange the egg whites on a pleasing plate and fill them with the combination. Garnish with the rest of the chives and bacon. You can end with a little fleur de sel and a touch extra truffle oil, if necessary. Calories: 125 kcal

Shrimp Tempura

Ingredients:

- 1/2 kg clean shrimp
- Garlic and salt to season shrimp
- 4 whole eggs
- 5 tablespoons of flour
- 1 Red Seasonal Envelope or Seasonal for FishOil for frying

Method of Preparation:

1. Season the smooth shrimp with garlic and salt and set aside. Beat whole eggs till soft, upload a pinch of Salt, the seasoning and flour, and beat appropriately with a fork until smooth.

2. Gradually dip the shrimp on this batter and fry in warm oil.

3. When browning the dough, take away with a slotted spoon and drain on an absorbent paper towel.

4. Serve warm as it tastes or maybe with white rice and shrimp sauce.

5. Enjoy your food.

Copycat Chilis Southwest Egg Rolls

Ingredients:

- 8 oz chicken breast
- 1 teaspoon of olive oil vegetable oil is fine 1 tablespoon of olive oil vegetable oil is fine 1/4 cup chopped red bell pepper
- 1/4 cup chopped spring onions - 1/2 cup of frozen corn
- 1/2 cup canned black beans, rinsed and drained 1/4 cup frozen spinach, thawed and drained
- 2 teaspoons of pickled jalapeno pepper, chopped 1 teaspoon of taco spice
- 3/4 cup of grated Monterey Jack cheese
- 8/7 inch flour tortillas
- 1/4 cup mashed fresh avocados (about half an avocado) 1 pack of Ranch Dressing Mix
- 1/2 cup milk - 1/2 cup mayonnaise - 2 tablespoons of chopped tomatoes
- 1 tablespoon of chopped onions

Instructions:

1. Season with salt and black pepper to the fowl. Brush the fowl breast with olive oil. Grill on a grill with medium heat. Cook on each side for five to 7 mins. Cut the hen into tiny pieces. Set apart the fowl.

2. Saute till tender red pepper. Refer to the aggregate of the green onion, rice, black beans, spinach, and pickled jalapenos. Attach the seasoning of taco. Via the sun.

3. Place the tortillas in the same quantities of the filing, identical amounts of chicken, and pinnacle with cheese. Fold and roll-up on the ends of the tortilla. Make positive the tortillas are very tight to roll. To defend the pin with toothpicks.

4. We are growing enough vegetable oil in a big pot to cover the pan's backside through 4 inches. Heat up to 350°C. Deep fry the rolls of the eggs until golden brown. It ought to take seven to eight mins. When extracting golden from oil, growing it on a rack of wire.

5. Prepare a container of mayonnaise half-cup ranch dressing mix and buttermilk half of cup. Remove the aggregate 1/4 cup of mashed avocado. In a blender, pump the combination till the sauce is mixed.

Nutrition:

Calories: 502kcal Carbohydrates: 42 g Protein: 19 g Fat: 28 g Saturated fat: 7g Cholesterol: 46 mg Sodium: 1088 mg Potassium: 443 mg Fiber: 3 g Sugar: 4 g Vitamin A: 1190IU Vitamin C: 13,9 mg Calcium: 212 mg Iron: 3 mg

Classic Chicken Salad Sandwich

Whether for lunch or dinner, chicken salad sandwiches are always a success in my family gatherings. Serve them for lunch and enjoy them with slices of tomatoes or chips. You can also make them part of a sandwich dinner with fries and mixed salad. To make this classic chicken salad sandwich recipe, you can use leftover chicken or purchased roast chicken and even bake or boil two or three chicken supremes.

Ingredients:

- 1½ cups cooked and chopped chicken
- 3 tablespoons finely chopped onion
- ¼ cup finely chopped celery
- 1 large hard and chopped egg
- 1 tablespoon dill sauce
- ½ cup of mayonnaise
- ¼ teaspoon salt
- 1/8 teaspoon ground black pepper
- 8 slices of bread

Step by step elaboration:

1. Gather all the ingredients inside the chicken salad sandwich and feature them on hand.

2. In a medium bowl, integrate cooked, chopped fowl, onion, celery, and egg; Stir to combine.

3. Add dill sauce, mayonnaise, salt, and floor black pepper. Mix all the components correctly, and if you need to moisten the education even extra, you can add a little more excellent mayonnaise.

4. Place a leaf of lettuce on every slice of bread and positioned one or tablespoons of the chicken aggregate on the pinnacle.

Ham and cheese grinders

The pinwheels ham and cheese are incredibly easy to make snacks and processed in a short time. Also, you will only need eight ingredients. You can store them in the refrigerator for a few days and reheat them just before the party. Adults and children will really enjoy these exquisite, crispy and salty snacks.

Ingredients:

- 300 g of refrigerated pizza dough - 2 cloves of garlic
- 2 tablespoons olive oil
- 1 teaspoon Italian seasoning
- ¼ cup grated Parmesan cheese
- 1 cup shredded mozzarella cheese
- 250 g sliced ham
- 1 egg
- Chopped fresh parsley
- Marinara sauce

Step by step elaboration:

1. Gather all of the elements to make ham and cheese grinders.

2. Preheat the oven to 180 ° C. Add the chopped garlic and the Italian seasoning to the olive oil.

3. Spread the chilled pizza dough in a large rectangle and reduce the choppy edges if desired.

4. Distribute the olive oil combination over the dough and sprinkle the grated Parmesan cheese and 1/2 of the grated mozzarella cheese over the dough floor.

5. Cowl the surface of the cheese with cooked ham and sprinkle the surface with the rest of the grated mozzarella cheese. Roll the dough as you could see inside the image.

6. Seal the edges of the dough through becoming a member of the dough and cut into nine parts. Place the ham and cheese grinders on a baking sheet lined with parchment paper.

7. Beat the egg with a teaspoon of warm water until well mixed.

Brush the egg on the top and sides of the grinders.

8. Bake the grinders for 15 to twenty minutes or till they're fluffy and golden brown.

9. Cover the grinders with chopped fresh parsley and serve right away with marinara sauce.

Mozzarella cheese sticks recipe

The mozzarella cheese sticks are coated with a simple breaded and quickly fried in hot oil until golden brown. Try to make this easy recipe and dip them in marinara sauce or pizza sauce. I assure you that they are exquisite snacks that nobody can resist!

Ingredients:

- ¼ cup flour
- 1 cup breadcrumbs
- 2 eggs
- 1 tablespoon milk
- 500 g mozzarella cheese
- 1 cup of vegetable oil
- 1 cup marinara sauce

Step by step elaboration:

1. Gather all of the elements of mozzarella cheese sticks.

2. Beat eggs and milk together in a medium bowl.

3. Cut the mozzarella into sticks 2 x 2 cm thick.

4. Cover each mozzarella cane with flour. Then dip them inside the egg and then within the breadcrumbs.

5. Dip the mozzarella sticks lower back into the egg and skip them in breadcrumbs.

6. Take to the freezer earlier than frying.

7. Heat the oil within the pan and prepare dinner the mozzarella cheese sticks for approximately a minute on every aspect or until well browned.

8. Drain the cheese sticks on paper napkins and serve with marinara sauce or pizza sauce.

Copycat Mac and Cheese with Smoked Gouda Cheese and Pumpkin

Ingredients:

- 1 1/2 tbsp olive oil
- 120 grams of fresh baguette torn into small pieces 2 teaspoons fresh thyme leaves
- 1/4 cup grated Parmesan
- 450 grams of spiral pasta (or penne)
- 4 tablespoons salted butter
- 4 tablespoons of flour
- 3 cups of whole milk at room temperature
- 1 cup canned pumpkin puree
- 2 cups smoked and chopped gouda cheese
- 2 cups cut sharp cheddar
- Kosher Salt

How to make:

1. Preheat oven to 190°C. Grease a large pan with nonstick cooking spray.

2. In a massive bowl, combine the cornbread, olive oil, thyme, and ½ tsp kosher Salt. Put in greased pan and bake till golden brown (12 to 15 minutes). Remove from oven, incorporate grated Parmesan and set aside.

3. In a large pan of boiling salted water, cook the pasta al dente in line with package deal directions. Drain the water and set aside the pasta.

4. Melt the butter in a large casserole over medium heat.

Incorporate the flour and cook dinner, continually stirring, till the aggregate starts to thicken (about one to mins).

5. Gradually include the milk, continually mixing until it paperwork a lightly thickened sauce (five to six minutes).

6. Add the mashed pumpkin and two teaspoons of kosher salt. Beat till included adequately into the sauce.

7. Lower the warmth and location, the gouda and cheddar cheeses, mixing nicely until melted.

8. Incorporate the cooked pasta into the sauce. Transfer the whole lot to a prepared baking sheet.

9. Sprinkle with toasted breadcrumbs. Put in oven and let till golden and blistered (about 20 mins). Serve immediately.

Baked Buffalo Meatballs

Ingredients:

- 350 gram of ground chicken meat
- 1 clove of minced garlic
- 1/4 cup of ground bread
- 2 tablespoons grated parmesan
- 2 teaspoons fresh celery leaves
- 1 egg
- 1/4 cup flour
- salt and pepper to taste
- 1/2 cup botanica sauce (Valentina or buffalo botanica) 2 tablespoons melted butter
- 1 tablespoon apple cider
- vinegar
- garlic powder and celery salt to taste for blue cheese dressing 1/3 cup of mayonnaise
- 1/3 cup sour cream
- 1 tablespoon lemon juice
- 1/4 cup blue cheese salt and pepper to taste

Directions:

1. Preheat the oven to 190°C

2. Mix the chook with the garlic, the ground bread, the Parmesan, the celery, the egg, and the flour; salpimenta

3. Form balls together with your arms and region them on a tray with foil; bake for 18 mins

4. Mix the botanica sauce with the melted butter and season with garlic powder and celery salt, bathe on this sauce every meatball as quickly as they go away the oven

5. To make the dressing, blend the cream, mayonnaise, lemon and half of the blue cheese; upload the relaxation of the crumbled cheese and season to taste

6. Serve the meatballs with chopsticks observed via blue cheese dressing.

Air Fryer ham and cheese sales

Ingredients:

- 1 tube of chilled pizza crust
- 1/4 pound Black Forest deli ham cut into thin slices 1 medium-sized pear, cut into thin slices and divided 1/4 cup of chopped walnuts, toasted
- 2 tablespoons of crumbled blue cheese

Instructions:

1. Preheat the fryer to 400 °. Unroll the pizza crust in a 12-in on a lightly floured surface. Square, rectangular. Split into four squares. Layer ham, half of the pear slices, walnuts, and blue cheese are diagonally higher than half of every square to 1/2 in.

Of the rims. Fold one nook to the other corner over filling, forming a triangle; force the edges to seal with a fork.

2. Arrange turnovers in greased air-fryer basket in batches in a single layer; spritz with cooking spray. Cook for a few minutes on each side till golden brown. Garnish with the relaxation of the slices.

Nutrition:

1 conversion: 357 calories, 10 g fat (2 g saturated fat), 16 mg cholesterol, 885mg sodium, 55 g carbohydrates (11 g sugar, 3 g fiber), 15 g protein.

Ham and Cheese Empanadas Recipe

If you love ham and cheese empanadas, but for fear that they explode in the oven, you avoid making them and, therefore, you end up ordering delivery, then I bring you a recipe with some tricks that will be extremely useful when preparing them in House. Let's go for the list of ingredients and the elaboration step by step!

Ingredients:

- 12 cooked ham fetas
- 400 g mozzarella cheese
- 12 empanada tapas
- Dried oregano
- Ground chili pepper
- 1 beaten egg

Step by step elaboration:

1. Cut the mozzarella cheese into 12 bars of approximately 30-35 g each.

2. Pass the bars with oregano and floor chili pepper and area them in the center of each ham feta.

3. Wrap the cheese with the ham, forming a bundle and reserve.

This is so that the cheese does no longer explode in the oven or while you're frying them.

4. Stretch the dough of the empanadas a touch so that they're oval and location the applications of ham and cheese in the center of each one in all them.

5. Close the middle and location a finger inside to push the ham even as persevering with to close the sides. This is so that the ham does not complicate your existence at the time of creating the repulgue. Make the traditional repulgue and forestalls placed them in an appropriate greased baking sheet with oil.

6. Paint the pies ham and cheese with crushed egg if desired and takes a warm oven till their golden brown.

7. If you want to fry ham and cheese empanadas, consider that the oil must be at 150-160 ° C, because if it had been hotter, they would be cooked on the outside and inside the cheese could no longer melt. Fry them for about 3 minutes.

8. Remove the patties fried ham and cheese with a slotted spoon and depart them on paper towels to cast off extra oil.

LUNCH RECIPES

Chi-Chi Seafood Chimichanga

Servings: 6 servings

Nutrition: Carbohydrates: 77g/ Protein: 44g/ Fat: 33g

Ingredients:

- 1 package flour tortillas (6 or 8 inch)
- 1 package (16-ounce size) crab meat, flaked
- 1 cup cottage cheese
- 1/4 cup Parmesan cheese
- 1 egg
- 1 tablespoon dried parsley flakes
- 1/4 teaspoon onion powder
- 4 tablespoons butter or margarine
- 4 tablespoons flour
- 1/2 teaspoon salt
- 2 dashes black pepper
- 2 cups milk or evaporated skim milk
- 8 ounces grated Monterey Jack cheese
- 1 tablespoon lemon juice

Instructions:

1. Preheat oven to 375 degrees F.

2. Mix all ingredients besides tortillas. Warm tortillas until pliable (approximately 10 seconds in the microwave). Wet one aspect of tortilla and region wet aspect down. Spoon on filling ingredients. Roll to keep in filling.

3. Spray baking dish with nonstick coating. Lay chimichangas seam facet down on the baking dish. Bake 25 mins. Serve with cheese sauce.

4. For Cheese Sauce: In a small saucepan melt butter or margarine. Stir in flour, salt, and pepper. Add milk all at once. Cook and stir over medium heat until thickened and bubbly. Cook and stir 1 to 2 minutes more.

5. Remove from heat. Add cheese, stir until melted. Just earlier than serving, upload lemon juice and stir until smooth.

Panera cheese and spinach egg soufflé
Servings: 4 servings

Nutrition: Carbohydrates: 37g/ Protein: 15g/ Fat: 28g

Ingredients:

- 3 tablespoons frozen spinach, thawed - 3 tablespoons minced artichoke hearts
- 2 teaspoons minced onion - 1 teaspoon minced red bell pepper
- 5 eggs - 2 tablespoons milk - 2 tablespoons heavy cream
- 1/4 cup shredded cheddar cheese - 1/4 cup shredded Monterey Jack cheese
- 1 tablespoon shredded Parmesan cheese - 1/4 teaspoon salt
- 1 8-ounce tube Pillsbury Crescent butter flake dough Cooking spray
- 1/4 cup shredded Asiago cheese

Instructions:

1. Preheat oven to 375°F.

2. Combine spinach, artichoke hearts, onion, and purple bell pepper in a small bowl. Add 2 tablespoons of water, cover bowl with plastic wrap and poke a few holes inside the plastic—microwave on high for three mins.

3. Beat four eggs. Mix in milk, cream, cheddar cheese, Jack cheese, Parmesan, and salt. Stir in spinach, artichoke, onion, and bell pepper. Microwave egg aggregate for 30 seconds on high, and then stir it. Do this 4 to 5 more instances or until you have a very runny scrambled egg mixture. This procedure will tighten up the eggs sufficient so that the dough won't sink into the eggs while it's folded over.

4. Unroll and separate the crescent dough into four rectangles. Don't tear the dough along the perforations that make triangles. Instead, pinch the dough collectively alongside the ones diagonal perforations so you have 4 rectangles.

5. Use a few flours on the dough and roll throughout the width of the rectangle with a rolling pin so that each piece of dough stretches out right into a s q uare this is approximately 6 inches by way of 6 inches.

6. Spray four 4-inch baking dishes or ramekins with cooking spray. Line every ramekin with the dough, then spoon same amounts of egg combination into each ramekin.

7. Sprinkle 1 tablespoon of Asiago cheese on top of the egg combination in each ramekin, after which gently fold the dough over the combination. Beat the remaining egg in a small bowl, then brush beaten egg over the top of the dough in every ramekin.

8. Bake for 25 to a half-hour or till the dough is brown. Remove from oven and cool for five mins, then carefully dispose of the soufflés from every ramekin and serve hot.

Sonic's Super SONIC Copycat Burrito

Servings: 6 servings

Nutrition: Carbohydrates: 10g/ Protein: 24g/ Fat: 50g

Ingredients:

- 1 1/2 cups Tater Tots
- 1 pound ground sausage
- 1/2 pound bacon
- 6 ounces American cheese
- 4 tablespoons milk, divided use
- 10 Eggs salt and pepper
- 1/2 cup shredded Cheddar cheese
- 1 jalapeno pepper slices
- 6 flour tortillas

Instructions:

1. Preheat the oven to 350 degrees. Spray a baking sheet with nonstick spray and location the Tater Tots on the baking sheet. Bake for about 22 to 25 minutes. While the little tater toddlers are in the oven, cook dinner the sausage in a skillet over medium warmness until it's far nicely browned. Drain sausage over paper towels and cover with every other paper towel to help keep the heat in as you still cook the breakfast.

2. You can cook the bacon within the same pan that you cooked the sausage in. Cook the bacon until crispy. Remove bacon from pan and drain on paper towels. Sonic serves their burrito with a cheese sauce. Cube the 6 oz of oz of American cheese and place in a small pot over low warmness and upload 2 tablespoons of milk. Melt the cheese, stirring fre q uently, the milk and cheese will combine to shape a cheese sauce. Once the cheese sauce has formed turn off the burner and leave the pot on the stovetop, the residual warmness will maintain the sauce fluid even as you prepare dinner the eggs.

3. In a medium-sized bowl, integrate the eggs with the final 2 tablespoons of milk. Spray a nonstick skillet with nonstick spray. Over medium warmth upload the egg and milk combination— Season eggs with a pinch of salt, and a pinch of black pepper. Gently stir the eggs as they prepare dinner. Once they may be done put off from the warmth. Heat tortillas for about 60 seconds to make them warm and pliable.

4. Assemble these using dispensing the eggs, sausage, tater children, bacon, and cheese sauce over the tortillas. If you want to upload some jalapeno slices to the burritos do so, in case you desire, upload a bit sprinkle of Cheddar cheese earlier than folding the burritos. If desired you can fold up the burritos, and wrap in plastic, and location inside the freezer so that you can reheat later.

Hot n 'Spicy Buffalo Wings by Hooters

Servings: 6 servings

Nutrition: Carbohydrates: 44g/ Protein: 44g/ Fat: 33g

Ingredients:

- 5 pounds chicken wings cut into two pieces 2 cups whole wheat flour
- 1 cup all purpose flour
- 2 1/2 teaspoons salt
- 1 teaspoon paprika
- 1/4 teaspoon cayenne pepper

Instructions:

1. In a large blending bowl, blend flours, salt, paprika and cayenne pepper, and blend nicely. Cut hen wings into drumettes and flappers. Wash and drain fowl. Coat bird in flour aggregate; refrigerate bird wings for 90 mins.

2. Cut hen wings into drumettes and flappers. Wash and drain fowl.

3. Coat hen in flour mixture; refrigerate chicken wings for 90 minutes.

4. When equipped to deep fry chicken wings, warm oil to 375 ranges. Place fowl pieces in heated oil, but do not crowd. Fry hen wings till golden brown. Remove from oil and drain.

5. When all wings have been fried, location in a massive bowl. Add Hot Sauce aggregate and mix thoroughly. Use a fork or tongs to vicinity hen portions on a serving platter. Serve right now and with plenty of paper towels.

Eggrolls of southwestern Chili

Servings: 5 servings

Nutrition: Carbohydrates: 21.8g/ Protein: 13.6g/ Fat: 31.2g

Ingredients:

- 2 tablespoons vegetable oil - 1 skinless, boneless chicken breast half
- 2 tablespoons minced green onion - 2 tablespoons minced red bell pepper
- ⅓ cup frozen corn kernels
- ¼ cup black beans, rinsed and drained
- 2 tablespoons frozen chopped spinach, thawed and drained 2 tablespoons diced jalapeno peppers
- ½ tablespoon minced fresh parsley - ½ teaspoon ground cumin
- ½ teaspoon chili powder - ⅓ teaspoon salt
- 1 pinch ground cayenne pepper
- ¾ cup shredded Monterey Jack cheese
- 5 (6 inch) flour tortillas
- 1 quart oil for deep frying

Instructions:

Rub 1 tablespoon vegetable oil over hen breast. In a medium saucepan over medium heat, cook bird about 5 minutes in step with side, till meat is now not pink and juices run clear. Remove from heat and set aside. Heat last 1 tablespoon vegetable oil in a medium saucepan over medium warmth. Stir in green onion and purple pepper. Cook and stir 5 minutes, till tender. Dice bird and mix into the pan with onion and pink pepper. Mix in corn, black beans, spinach, jalapeno peppers, parsley, cumin, chili powder, salt and cayenne pepper. Cook and stir five minutes, till properly mixed and tender. Remove from heat and stir in Monterey Jack cheese in order that it melts. Wrap tortillas with a clean, lightly wet cloth. Microwave on high approximately 1 minute, or till warm and pliable.

Spoon even quantities of the combination into every tortilla.

Fold ends of tortillas, then roll tightly around combination.

Secure with toothpicks. Arrange in a medium dish, cowl with plastic, and place in the freezer. Freeze as a minimum of 4 hours.

In a large, deep skillet, warmness oil for deep frying to 375 tiers F (a hundred ninety stages C). Deep fry frozen, stuffed tortillas 10 minutes every, or till darkish golden brown. Drain on paper towels earlier than serving.

Guacamole of Chipotle

Servings: 4 servings

Nutrition: Carbohydrates: 8.3g/ Protein: 1.7g/ Fat: 11.1g

Ingredients:

- 2 large Hass avocados halved and pitted 1 teaspoon fresh lemon juice
- 1 teaspoon fresh lime juice
- 1/4 cup red onion finely chopped
- 1/2 jalapeño chile stemmed, seeded, and finely chopped (see notes)
- 2 tablespoons cilantro leaves finely chopped
- salt

Tortilla chips for serving

Instructions:

1. In a medium bowl, combine avocados, lemon juice, and lime juice. Mash till smooth. Stir in onion, cilantro, and jalapeños season to taste with salt. Serve with chips.

2. To refrigerate, an area in a bowl and press plastic wrap directly on top of the entire floor of the guacamole, so no element is exposed to air.

Pesto Corkscrew by Noodles & Company

Servings:4 servings

Nutrition: Carbohydrates: 9.4g/ Protein: 28.6g/ Fat: 316g

Ingredients:

- 4 medium-large zucchini (about 2 pounds), trimmed ¾ teaspoon salt, divided
- 2 cups packed fresh basil leaves
- ¼ cup pine nuts, toasted
- ¼ cup grated Parmesan cheese
- 1/4 cup plus 2 tablespoons extra-virgin olive oil, divided 2 tablespoons lemon juice
- 1 large clove garlic, q uartered
- ½ teaspoon ground pepper
- 1 pound boneless, skinless chicken breast, cut into 1-inch pieces

Instructions:

1. Using a spiral vegetable slicer, reduce zucchini lengthwise into long, skinny strands. Give the strands a chop here and there so the noodles aren't too long. Place the zucchini in a colander and toss with 1/4 teaspoon salt. Let drain for 15 to 30 minutes, then gently squeeze to put off any excess liquid.

2. Meanwhile, vicinity basil, pine nuts, Parmesan, 1/4 cup oil, lemon juice, garlic, pepper, and 1/four teaspoon salt in a mini food processor. Process till nearly smooth.

3. Heat 1 tablespoon oil in a huge skillet over medium-high warmth. Add chicken in a single layer; sprinkle with the final 1/four teaspoon salt. Cook, stirring, till just cooked through, about 5 minutes. Transfer to a large bowl and stir in 3 tablespoons of the pesto.

4. Add the final 1 tablespoon oil to the pan. Add the drained zucchini noodles and toss lightly till warm, 2 to three minutes.

Transfer to the bowl with the chicken. Add the remaining pesto and toss gently to coat.

DINNER RECIPES

Cajun Chicken Pasta from Chili

Servings: 4 servings

Nutrition: Carbohydrates: 26g/ Protein: 28g/ Fat: 17.8g

Ingredients:

- 2 chicken breasts, boneless skinless - 4 teaspoons Cajun Seasoning
- 4 tablespoons butter or 4 tablespoons margarine 3 cups heavy cream
- ½ teaspoon lemon pepper seasoning
- 1 teaspoon salt - 1 teaspoon black pepper
- ¼ teaspoon garlic powder
- 8 ounces penne pasta, cooked and drained
- 2 Roma tomatoes, diced
- ½ cup parmesan cheese, fresh shredded, to taste

Instructions:

1. Slightly moisten chicken with water.

2. In a big resealable plastic bag, shake bird and cajun Seasoning till the bird is very well coated.

3. In a large skillet, saute hen in 2 tablespoons butter, over medium warmness, turning each time necessary.

4. When fowl is set half-way done, take hold of a 2nd skillet and combine heavy cream, 2 tablespoons butter, and the rest of seasonings over medium warmth, stirring occasionally.

5. When the cream mixture starts to bubble, upload the pasta and turn off the heat. Stir well.

6. When a bird is cooked through, a region on cutting board and slice into strips.

7. Spoon pasta and sauce onto huge serving plates (2) and pinnacle with the bird, diced tomatoes, and Parmesan.

8. Throw a thick, garlicky slice of Texas toast on that bad boy and enjoy!

Panda Express Chow Mein

Servings: 2 servings

Nutrition: Carbohydrates: 23g/ Protein: 4g/ Fat: 4g

Ingredients:

- 4 oz. fresh yaki-soba noodles
- 1/4 cup low sodium soy sauce
- 4 cloves garlic, minced
- 1 tbsp. brown sugar
- 2 tsp. ginger, minced
- 1/4 tsp. pepper
- 1 tbsp. olive oil
- 1 onion, diced
- 2 celery ribs, chopped
- 4 cups shredded cabbage

Instructions:

1. Prepare the yaki-soba noodles in line with the package instructions. Do no longer use a seasoning packing if included.

For fresh noodles, just add them to boiling water for 1-2 minutes till they separate and emerge as tender. Dried noodles usually need to be boiled for 4-5 minutes.

2. Meanwhile, mix together the soy sauce, brown sugar, ginger, garlic, and pepper.

3. Heat the olive oil over medium-high warmness, Add the onion and celery and cook dinner for 3-four minutes. Add the cabbage and cook for 2 minutes until simply tender. Add the noodles and the sauce. Cook for two-three mins, stirring often. Taste and season if wished with extra soy sauce or pepper.

Pasta with rattlesnake from Pizzeria Uno

Servings: 1 serving

Nutrition: Carbohydrates: 128g/ Protein: 58g/ Fat: 71g

Ingredients:

- 2 skinless, boneless chicken breast halves, cut into cubes
- 2 tablespoons butter
- 2 cloves garlic, minced
- 1 tablespoon Italian Seasoning
- 1 pound penne pasta
- 4 tablespoons butter
- 2 cloves garlic, minced
- 1/3 cup all-purpose flour
- 1 tablespoon salt
- 1/4 teaspoon ground white pepper
- 2 cups milk
- 1 cup half-and-half
- 3/4 cup grated Parmesan cheese
- 8 ounces shredded Colby-Monterey Jack cheese
- 1 (4 ounces) jar jalapeno peppers (in juice), sliced

Instructions:

1. In a large skillet over medium warmth, integrate chook, 2 tablespoons butter, garlic, and Italian Seasoning. Cook till hen is not pink inside. Remove from skillet and set aside.

2. Cook pasta for eight to 10 minutes; drain.

3. Meanwhile, begin making a roux: Melt four tablespoons butter in a skillet. Add garlic.

4. Stir in flour, salt and pepper; cook 2 minutes stirring constantly.

5. Slowly add milk and half-and-half, hold to stir till clean and creamy.

6. Stir in Parmesan and Colby-Monterey Jack cheeses; stir until the cheese is melted.

7. Add jalapeno peppers and stir in chicken.

8. Add Alfredo mixture to cooked penne pasta and serve.

Copycat Kung Pao Spaghetti from the California Pizza Kitchen

Servings: 6 servings

Nutrition: Carbohydrates: 129g/ Protein: 57g/ Fat: 44g

Ingredients:

- 1 1⁄2 cup chicken stock
- 2 tablespoons cornstarch
- 3⁄4 cup soy sauce
- 1⁄2 cup dry sherry
- 3 tablespoons red chili paste with garlic 1⁄4 cup sugar
- 2 tablespoons red wine vinegar
- 2 tablespoons toasted sesame oil
- 2 egg whites
- 2 tablespoons cornstarch
- 1⁄2 teaspoon salt
- 1 lb spaghetti
- 1⁄2 cup olive oil, plus
- 2 tablespoons olive oil
- 1 lb boneless skinless chicken breast, cut in 3/4-inch cubes 10 -15 whole chinese dried red chili peppers (don't eat these, they are for color and heat)
- 1 cup unsalted dry roasted peanuts
- 1⁄4 cup minced garlic
- 3 cups coarsely-chopped scallions, greens and whites

Instructions:

1. In a medium saucepan, whisk the fowl inventory and cornstarch collectively until the cornstarch is completely dissolved. Stir in all the closing sauce ingredients and convey to a boil over medium-high heat. Reduce the heat and simmer until the sauce is thick sufficient to coat the again of a spoon, 15 to twenty minutes. Set aside.

2. In a blending bowl, use a whisk to stir together the egg whites, cornstarch, and salt till thoroughly blended; be careful no longer to beat them into a foam. Set aside.

3. Bring a huge pot of salted water to a rapid boil. Add the pasta and prepare dinner till al dente, eight to 10 minutes.

4. Meanwhile, in a large nonstick frying pan over high heat, heat the olive oil for approximately 1 minute. Add the hen pieces to the Egg White-Cornstarch Mixture and toss to coat them. Taking care to avoid splattering, add the coated bird to the pan and cook dinner like a stable pancake till the egg aggregate sets; then, the use of a large spatula, cautiously turn the fowl pieces over together and, with a wood spoon, gently separate the pieces.

5. Gently stir the Chinese peppers and roasted peanuts into the pan.

As quickly as they darken in color, after no more than 1 minute, stir inside the garlic and scallions. Once the garlic starts to brown, after no extra than 30 seconds, upload the Kung Pao Sauce and toss and stir to coat the ingredients.

6. When the pasta is prepared, drain it nicely and, in a big mixing or serving bowl, toss it very well with the sauce. Serve family-fashion or transfer to individual serving bowls, arranging the chicken, vegetables, and peppers.

Three Applebee Cheese Chicken Penne

Servings: 4 servings

Nutrition: Carbohydrates: 91g/ Protein: 57g/ Fat: 46g

Ingredients:

- 1 teaspoon fresh basil leaf ; sliced thin
- 2 small roma tomatoes ; diced
- 1 garlic clove ; pressed
- 1/4 teaspoon salt - 1/2 teaspoon olive oil
- 1 lb chicken breast
- 2 tablespoons lemon juice
- 1 tablespoon olive oil - 1/2 teaspoon Italian spices
- 5 button mushrooms; sliced
- 1 tablespoon purple onion; very thin sliced (optional) 1 jar roasted garlic alfredo sauce
- 2 ounces provolone cheese; shredded or chopped small 2 ounces grated parmesan cheese
- 2 ounces mozzarella cheese; chopped small or shredded 2 teaspoons olive oil
- 1/2 pound penne pasta; according to to box directions

Instructions:

1. 2T lemon juice, 1 T olive oil and Italian seasonings together, pour over chicken and place in a plastic bag or a marinator container. (i exploit a vacuume sealed container to hurry up process) allow, marinate for 30 minutes to some hours.

2. Start bruschetta aggregate too. Just blend all together and cover in the fridge until dinner is prepared to serve.

3. Heat grill and cook dinner chicken on a medium warmness until the bird is done. Start to prepare dinner your pasta on the stove according to package instructions.

4. Meanwhile warmth 2 tsp olive oil over med-high heat in a heavy skillet and cook mushrooms and onions till tender. Flip off empty skillet jar of alfredo sauce into the skillet and add drained cooked pasta.

5. Chook is done. Slice thick or thin and upload to the skillet blend altogether.

6. Heat contents of skillet up until pretty much bubbly then upload the cheeses and mix appropriately until mixed and melted.

7. Serve in pasta dishes and top with bruschetta mix along with some garlic bread or sticks that are a great meal!

Boston Market Mac n 'Cheese

Servings: 8 servings

Nutrition: Carbohydrates: 34g/ Protein: 17g/ Fat: 29g

Ingredients:

- 8 tablespoons butter unsalted (1 stick)
- 1/2 cup flour
- 1 teaspoon salt
- 1/4 teaspoon black pepper
- 1/2 teaspoon dry mustard
- 4 cups milk whole
- 8 ounces American cheese
- 1/2 cup blue cheese
- 1/2 cup cheddar cheese
- 8 ounces semolina rotini pasta cooked

Instructions:

1. Heat the oven to four hundred degrees.

2. Melt the butter on medium warmth, then add in the flour, salt, pepper, and mustard.

3. Whisk until clean and prepare dinner for 30 seconds.

4. Add in the milk slowly in 1 cup increments until smooth.

5. Add in the cheese and whisk till wholly melted.

6. Add within the pasta and stir.

7. Pour into a baking dish and bake, including for 20 mins 22.

Macaroni Grill's Pasta Milano

Servings: 8 servings

Nutrition: Carbohydrates: 67g/ Protein: 30g/ Fat: 10g

Ingredients:

- 6 ounces butter
- 18 ounces grilled chicken, sliced 12 ounces sun-dried tomatoes
- 12 ounces mushrooms, sliced
- 6 tablespoons finely grated parmesan cheese
- 36 ounces roasted garlic cream sauce - recipe below 36 ounces bow tie pasta
- 2 cups heavy cream
- 2 tablespoons chopped garlic
- Dash salt & pepper
- 1 teaspoons beef base or 1 beef bouillon cube
- 1 tablespoon butter

Instructions:

1. Make the sauce, and guidelines are below.

2. Cook the pasta as directed on the package.

3. Sauté butter and mushrooms for approximately 30 seconds. Add the roasted garlic cream sauce and Parmesan; warmness thoroughly.

4. Drain pasta. Add pasta to the sauté pan and mix nicely. Add the sliced and cooked chicken, and the chopped sun-dried tomatoes.

5. Garnish with Parmesan cheese. Serve and enjoy.

PASTAS AND SALAD

Simple copycat Pizza Hut Cavatina

Ingredients:

- Cut 1/2 pound peppers into thin slices
- 1/4 pound spiral pasta
- 1 green pepper cut
- 1/4 pound Shell noodles
- Cut 1 onion into thin slices
- 1/4 pound of pasta
- 8 ounces of grated mozzarella
- 1/2 pound of hamburger browned
- 8 ounces of grated parmesan
- 1/2 pound Italian sausage browned
- 32 ounces of spaghetti sauce

Instructions:

1. Cook noodles inside the course of the packet. Heat the sauce and mix it with the hamburger and the sausage fried. Sprinkled with Pam cooking spray, layer noodles, and sauce in a pan of 11 X

2. for about forty-five mins at 350 stages or until the cheese is melted.

Nutrition: Calories: 467kcal Carbohydrates: 36 g Protein: 24 g Fat: 24 g Saturated fat: 10 g Sodium: 1384 mg Potassium: 487 mg Fiber: 2 g Sugar: 5 g Vitamin A: 640IU Vitamin C: 14 mg Calcium: 376 mg Iron: 2.6 mg

Spaghetti Pizza Recipe

This spaghetti pizza recipe is straightforward to make, but it takes a little while. However, it is worth it. It is a delicious and comforting dish and also has ground meat. Serve with a salad of green leaves and tomatoes and some toasted garlic bread. Let's go for the ingredient list and step by step!

Ingredients:

- 750 ml of pasta sauce - 500 g ground beef
- 500 g of spaghetti
- 400 g of tomatoes cut into small cubes
- 150 g sliced pepperoni
- 1 ½ cups shredded cheddar cheese
- 1 cup shredded Swiss cheese
- ½ cup grated Parmesan cheese
- ½ cup whole milk - 1 chopped onion
- 3 cloves garlic, minced
- 2 chopped red or green peppers
- 1 teaspoon dried Italian seasoning
- 2 large eggs

Directions:

1. Gather the ingredients to make the spaghetti pizza.

2. Preheat the oven to 170 ° C. Boil a big pot of water to cook dinner the spaghetti.

3. Cook the beef, chopped onion, chopped garlic, and chopped red and inexperienced peppers in a pan over medium warmness with oil until the beef is browned.

4. Drain properly and upload the pasta sauce, the tomatoes reduce into small cubes and the Italian seasoning. Stir properly and boil over medium warmness at the same time as getting ready spaghetti.

5. Cook the spaghetti according to the bundle instructions.

6. Combine the milk, eggs, and grated Parmesan cheese in a massive bowl and beat till mixed.

7. Strain the spaghetti and stir with the egg aggregate. Spread half of the spaghetti, egg, and milk mixture in a refractory dish and copper with half of the sauce and red meat combination. Repeat the layers. Bake in a preheated oven for 30 or 40 mins until hot and cowl with the closing cheeses, after which the pepperoni. Return to the oven and bake until the cheeses melt. Let stand for 5 minutes and reduce into squares to serve the spaghetti pizza.

Garden spaghetti carbonara

Ingredients:

- 1/4 cup of flour
- 1/4 cup butter
- 1 liter of milk
- 1/8 teaspoon of pepper
- 1/2 teaspoon of salt
- 18 oz bacon cut extra thick
- 1/4 cup of olive oil
- 12 oz sliced mushrooms
- 6 tablespoons of chopped shallots
- Cook 1 pound spaghetti according to the package insert 2 teaspoons of finely chopped parsley
- 1/2 cup grated parmesan cheese
- 2 ounces of freshly grated Fontina cheese

Instructions:

1. Melt butter over medium warmness in a 4-quarter robust casserole.

2. Remove the meal and prepare dinner for 1 minute. Add milk, salt, and pepper and stir vigorously with a wire whip till slightly boiling the mixture. Reduce warmth and boil for 5 mins even as the sauce thickens. Stir inside the sauce the Fontina cheese and allow it to soften inside the sauce. Stay warm.

3. Thoroughly prepare dinner the bacon. Drain on towels made of paper. Cut into pieces of 1/4-inch and whisk within the sauce. In a large skillet, soften olive oil over medium heat. Attach sliced onions and chopped mushrooms and saute till golden; attach to the sauce. Cook spaghetti within the direction of the box. Drain properly and add the parsley to the sauce. Mix properly and skip to a serving table. Sprinkle with Parmesan cheese and function quickly as possible.

Nutrition: Calories: 729kcal Carbohydrates: 52 g Protein: 23 g Fat: 46 g Saturated fat: 17 g Cholesterol: 82 mg Sodium: 425 mg Potassium: 438 mg Fiber: 2 g Sugar: 7 g Vitamin A: 555IU Vitamin C: 0.8 mg Calcium: 262 mg Iron: 1.4mg

Spaghetti Frittata

Frittatas are merely more resistant and easy to cook tortillas. They are one of the best quick recipes to prepare for brunch, breakfast, lunch, or dinner. The only rules for making frittata are to make sure that the eggs are well beaten and that the ingredients you add are well cooked before incorporating them.

Only then can you succeed. You can use almost any leftover food such as rice, pasta, diced potatoes, grilled meat, or vegetables. This time I will teach you how to make a spaghetti frittata step by step. Take note!

Ingredients:

- ½ cup chopped green pepper or ½ cup chopped onion 2 tablespoons olive oil
- 1 tablespoon butter
- ¼ cup milk
- 2 cups grated Parmesan cheese
- ½ teaspoon dried basil leaves
- 1 cup cooked spaghetti or fettuccine cut into 5 cm pieces 6 eggs

Direction:

1. Heat the olive oil and butter in a pan till it melts.

2. Add the green pepper and cook dinner over medium heat, frequently stirring until soft and crispy at the identical time.

3. Meanwhile, in a big bowl, mix the eggs with the milk, ¼ cup grated Parmesan cheese, salt and pepper, and basil.

4. Add the cooked pasta to the egg combination and stir gently.

5. Next, upload the egg combination to the pan and arrange the pasta in a uniform layer.

6. Cook the egg combination over medium warmness, raising the edges with a spatula now and then so that the uncooked egg flows underneath.

7. When the egg aggregate is nearly ready, but still moist, after 10 minutes, cover it with grated Parmesan cheese. Cook for a few more mins until it starts to brown. Remove from the oven and cut the spaghetti frittata into portions. Serve immediately.

Chopped Chicken Salad

What you need:

- 4 very compact cups of chopped romaine lettuce 2 very small cups of chicory (radicchio) chopped 2 cups cooked and chopped chicken
- 1 cup ditalini pasta (thimbles), cooked and rinsed 8 slices of hard salami OSCAR MAYER Hard Salami, chopped 4 ounces (1/2 pcs. Of 8 oz) of asiago cheese CRACKER
- BARREL Asiago Cheese, chopped
- 3/4 cup Italian dressing 'from the house' Tuscan style KRAFT
- Tuscan House Italian Dressing

Cooking tips:

1. This salad not simplest satisfies. However it also can be prepared in advance. Refrigerate for up to two hours earlier than serving.

2. Prepare it with robust salami with ground black pepper OSCAR

MAYER Cracked Black Pepper Hard Salami.

Nutrition: Calories: 648kcal Carbohydrate: 37 g Protein: 23 g Fat: 44 g Saturated fat: 10g Cholesterol: 85 mg Sodium: 761 mg Potassium: 482 mg Fiber: 2 g Sugar:13 g Vitamin A: 1015IU Vitamin C: 10.5 mg Calcium: 124 mg Iron: 1.8 mg

Omelet noodles

The noodle tortilla is a straightforward recipe to make that can be prepared even with the noodles leftover. If you don't have noodles, you can use any type of unfilled pasta that you like. This is an excellent recipe for use, of Italian origin. I hope you are encouraged to prepare it. I assure you you'll love it!

Ingredients:

- 200g noodles
- 6 eggs
- Fried Tomato Sauce
- Oregano
- Basil
- Salt and ground black pepper Olive oil
- Grated Parmesan cheese c / n

Direction:

1. Fill a pot with lots of water and pour a handful of salt.

2. Bring to heat, and while it boils, upload the pasta.

3. Stir with a wooden spoon sometimes and cook dinner al dente.

4. Drain the pasta while it's miles al dente and move through cold water to reduce the cooking.

5. Shell eggs and pepper.

6. Beat them with a twine whisk and add the noodles.

7. Pour a few oil right into a pan and produce it to the fire.

8. Divide the noodle aggregate into bowls and pour one into the pan. Cook over low heat so that it settles slowly.

9. Distribute the tomato sauce with the herbs on a pinnacle as if you had been making a pizza.

10. Sprinkle with cheese and pour the other combination of the eggs with the noodles on the pinnacle.

11. Help yourself with a spatula to cover the surface adequately and let it take a seat for a few mins.

12. Turn with the help of a plate about two or three times and pass shaping with the spatula even as cooking.

Cajun mimic Popeye recipe

Ingredients:

- 3 tablespoons of olive oil
- 1 teaspoon of sea salt
- 1 teaspoon of freshly ground black pepper
- 1 teaspoon of chili powder
- 1 teaspoon of garlic powder
- 1 teaspoon of brown sugar
- 1 teaspoon of paprika
- 1 teaspoon of oregano
- 1 teaspoon of cayenne pepper
- 1 teaspoon of onion powder
- 3 rusty potatoes

Instructions:

1. In a meals processor, finely chop or pulse the bird gizzards. Stir in ground beef, ground chook gizzards, bell pepper, and cook dinner over medium-high warmth until beef loses its pink color and soft bell pepper. Replace the grease excess.

2. Switch to medium or medium-low temperature. Remove remaining ingredients, stir and cook dinner until the ground pork is fully cooked, and about 25-35 mins of liquid are gone. For this Cajun at Heart, extra Creole Seasoning And Red Pepper Can Be Added.

Nutrition:

Calories: 350kcal Carbohydrates: 60 g Protein: 17 g Fat: 3 g Saturated fat: 1g Sodium: 52 mg Potassium: 292 mg Fiber: 1 g Sugar: 0 g Vitamin A: 370IU Vitamin C: 11.2 mg Calcium: 29 mg Iron: 2.1 mg

Eggplant cannelloni

Ingredients:

- 250g hake fillets without skin or bones
- 250g shrimp tails
- 50g grated cheese
- 2 medium eggplants 1 pack of cannelloni
- 1 tablet of chicken broth
- Bechamel sauce
- 2 bell peppers
- ½ liter of milk

Direction:

1. Wash the eggplants and reduce them lengthwise. Place them on a baking sheet and sprinkle with a drizzle of oil.

2. Bake the eggplants at 200 ° C for 20 mins.

3. Soak the cannelloni, and when they are nicely hydrated, get rid of them and dry them with a cloth.

4. Sauté the fish and prawns with a drizzle of oil and season with the bird stock.

5. Chop hake fillets, prawns, peppers, and the pulp of the eggplants you have got roasted. Mix with tablespoons of béchamel sauce and fill the cannelloni.

6. Place the eggplant cannelloni on a tray and cowl with béchamel sauce. Sprinkle grated cheese on top and gratin.

Pasta with mushrooms

The penne is a type of pasta of Italian origin, prepared from durum wheat.

Generally, they are available in the form of a dry paste, with a cylindrical shape cut obliquely at the ends and grooves on the outside. This type of pasta is called penne rigate, but if you don't have those lines on the outside, your name would be penne lisce . There is a wide variety of dishes with which you can use this pasta, and then I will teach you to create a paste with edible mushrooms and cherry tomatoes. Exquisite!

Ingredients:

- Penne 360g
- 250g cherry tomatoes
- 250g mushrooms
- 5g chopped fresh parsley
- 3 scallions
- 1 onion
- 1 tablespoon mustard
- 2 tablespoons olive, sunflower or corn oil 200 cm^3 of cream or milk cream

Direction:

1. Place plenty of water in a pot alongside a touch oil and salt.

Cook the pasta al dente and drain.

2. Cut the green onions into thin slices in addition to the fit to be eaten mushrooms. Cut the cherry tomatoes in half of and the onion in pen. Sauté the scallions and the commonplace onion in a nonstick skillet with a little oil and when the onion is translucent, add the mushrooms and cook dinner until golden brown.

3. Mix the cream or milk cream with the mustard and warmth in a pot. Add the cherry tomatoes to the pan, which you had to reduce in half of and, finally, add the cooked and drained pasta in conjunction with the onions.

4. Heat for some seconds and serve in dishes.

5. Garnish with chopped fresh parsley and room to flavor.

Green salad with Chicken Rey and egg

Ingredients:

- 1/2 iceberg lettuce
- 2 carrots
- 2 hard-boiled eggs
- 1 chicken breast
- 1 tomato Mayonnaise
- olive oil
- Pepper Salt

Preparation:

1. Wash and reduce the iceberg lettuce to Juliana. We booked in a big bowl.

2. We wash and cut the tomato into dice. We upload it to the bowl.

3. Peel and reduce the carrot julienne. We add to the bowl.

4. Cut the bird breast into strips.

5. Cook the eggs for 10-15 mins in a saucepan with a circulation of vinegar and salt, so that they do no longer break.

6. When the eggs are ready, we cast off, chill with a jet of water and take away the shell.

7. Chop the hard-boiled eggs into quarters and add to the bowl.

Meanwhile, in a pan with a drizzle of oil, location the fowl strips, season and brown the hen for five mins over medium warmness. Mix the salad with multiple tablespoons of mayonnaise to taste and serve immediately.

Nutrition:

Calories: 438kcal Carbohydrate: 5 g Protein: 19 g Fat: 36 g Saturated fat: 8 g Cholesterol: 571 mg Sodium: 1036 mg Potassium: 189 mg Fiber: 0 g Sugar: 5 g Vitamin A: 935IU Calcium: 75 mg Iron: 1.9 mg

Panera Bread Green Goddess Cobb Salad

Ingredients:

- 1 cup of sliced red onion
- 1/2 cup white vinegar
- 1 tablespoon of sugar
- 1 1/2 teaspoon of salt
- 1 cup of warm water Salad servers:
- 6 ounces of salad mix-use rocket, romaine, kale, and radicchio mix
- 6 ounces of grilled chicken breast
- 2 tablespoons of crispy cooked bacon
- 3 tablespoons of chopped avocado
- 1/2 cup of chopped tomatoes
- Halve 1 hard-boiled egg
- 2 tablespoons of feta
- 2 tablespoons of pickled onions Green goddess salad dressing: 1 cup of mayonnaise
- 2 tablespoons of tarragon leaves
- 3 tablespoons of chopped chives
- 1 cup of flat-leaf parsley
- 1 cup of packed watercress cleaned and hard stems removed 2 tablespoons of lemon juice
- 1 tablespoon of champagne vinegar - 1/2 teaspoon of salt
- 1/4 teaspoon of pepper

Direction:

1. Cut onions as thin as possible, I like to use the 1/eight inch putting on my mandolin. Put the onions in a jar full. Mix white vinegar, sugar, salt, and warm water in a small bowl. Stir till sugar and salt have dissolved. These should rest for an approximate half-hour for use. Put all the ingredients for the dressing within the bowl of a blender or meals processor and mix for 30-45 seconds, or until the dressing is mostly clean and creamy.

2. Place the salad on the bottom of a large salad bowl. Cut the fowl breast into thin slices and place them at the salad. Add bacon, chopped avocado, chopped tomatoes, feta cheese, hard-boiled egg halves, and pickled onions. Drizzle with as plenty of salad dressing as desired. Remaining salad dressing can be stored in an airtight box for 1 week.

Nutrition: Calories: 1175kcal Carbohydrate: 30 g Protein: 32 g Fat: 102 g Saturated fat: 19 g Cholesterol: 219 mg Sodium: 3603 mg Potassium: 1320 mg Fiber: 5 g Sugar: 15 g Vitamin A: 4930IU Vitamin C: 94.5 mg Calcium: 295 mg Iron: 6.5 mg

Caprese tomato, Mozzarella, Basil and Avocado Salad Récipe

Ingredients:

- 2 sliced avocados
- 2 ripe tomatoes
- 500 g mozzarella cheese
- 1 cup fresh basil leaves
- 1/4 cup olive oil
- 1/4 cup balsamic Aceto
- Salt and ground black pepper

Direction:

1. Gather all the ingredients to make this tomato, mozzarella, basil, and avocado Caprese salad.

2. With a small knife, cut the give up of the tomato stem and then, the use of a serrated knife, reduce the tomatoes into slices.

3. Cut the mozzarella into slices and spot alternating slices of avocado, tomato, mozzarella, and basil leaves in character dishes. Sprinkle with olive oil and balsamic vinegar and season gently with salt and ground black pepper.

4. Spread your Italian tomato, mozzarella, basil, and avocado salad with a fresh baguette or on a bed of romaine lettuce.

Creamy Potato Salad

If you are looking for a delicious and easy to make a side dish, this time we bring you a creamy potato salad. Dijon mustard and lemon juice balance its creamy flavor and make it even tastier. Prepare it at any time of the year and consent to all your family and friends at dinner time. Take note of the list of ingredients and elaboration step by step!

Ingredients:

- 1 kilo of potatoes
- ¾ cups of low-fat sour cream
- ¼ cup of mayonnaise
- ¼ cup chopped fresh parsley 3 tablespoons lemon juice 2 tablespoons Dijon mustard
- 2 tablespoons chopped fresh tarragon
- 2 chopped celery stalks
- 2 hard-boiled eggs
- 1 small fennel, thinly sliced

Direction:

1. Peel the potatoes and reduce them into medium cubes. Place them in a large pot with cold water and kosher salt to taste, and upload a touch salt. Bring to the fire, and while it boils, simmers until the potatoes are smooth 10 to 12 mins.

2. Mix mayonnaise with sour cream, mustard, and lemon juice.

3. Season with salt and ground black pepper and add heat potatoes.

Mix and allow cooling to room temperature.

4. Add the celery reduce into thin slices as well as fennel and parsley and tarragon, all finely chopped.

5. Mix so that the potatoes are impregnated with cream and add the hard-cut eggs in wedges. Serve the creamy potato salad.

Wedge Salad with Creamy Dressing

Ingredients:

- 1 cup Daisy Cream
- 1/2 cup skim milk
- 4 teaspoons cider vinegar
- 1 sachet of green onion powder mix
- 1 clove garlic, minced
- 1/2 cup sliced green onion
- 1 head of iceberg lettuce, removed the heart and in pictures 1 tomato, diced
- 4 teaspoons diced bacon

Instructions:

1. In a small bowl, combine the cream, buttermilk, vinegar and dressing mix. Beat till the combination is easy.

2. Add garlic and 1/four cup inexperienced onion; set aside.

Remove the middle of the lettuce and cut into 4 same wedges.

3. Place every wedge in 4 different dishes. Pour approximately 1/four of the salad dressing over every wedge.

4. Distribute 1/four of the ultimate onion, 1/4 of the chopped tomato, and 1 teaspoon of diced bacon on top of every wedge.

Tomatoes stuffed with tuna

Ingredients:

- 2 cans of water or natural tuna
- 4 medium tomatoes
- a large cup of white or brown rice
- Mayonnaise c / n
- Green olives c / n
- Peas or capers c / n
- 2 carrots
- Salt c / n

Direction:

1. Place masses of water in a pot and produce it to the fireplace.

When it boils, pour the rice. Stir with a timber spoon so that it does now not stick and prepare dinner for 20 minutes or until it's far soft. Remove, drain without delay, and reserve within the fridge.

2. Peel the carrots and cut them into small cubes. Cook in a pot with water until they soften. Drain and region in a bowl.

3. Add the rice, the two cans of drained tuna, the peas or capers (cooked), and the mayonnaise to taste.

4. Mix everything very well and room to taste.

5. Wash the tomatoes thoroughly and smoke them with the help of a knife and a spoon.

6. If you want to take gain of what you've got chosen to the tomato, reduce it into small cubes and blend it with the rice or save it for any other recipe.

7. Fill the tomatoes with the rice and the tuna. Garnish with some mayonnaise within the center and a green olive.

PIZZA AND SALAD RECIPES

Copycat California Pizza Kitchen California Club Pizza

Servings: 4 servings

Nutrition: Carbohydrates: 59g/ Protein: 29g/ Fat: 30g

Ingredients:

- 1 tablespoon cornmeal
- 1 loaf (1 pound) frozen pizza dough, thawed
- 1 cup shredded mozzarella cheese
- 1 cup ready-to-use grilled chicken breast strips 4 bacon strips, cooked and crumbled
- 2 cups shredded romaine
- 1 cup fresh arugula
- 1/4 cup mayonnaise
- 1 tablespoon lemon juice
- 1 teaspoon grated lemon zest
- 1/2 teaspoon pepper
- 1 medium tomato, thinly sliced
- 1 medium ripe avocado, peeled and sliced
- 1/4 cup loosely packed basil leaves, chopped

Instructions:

1. Preheat oven to 450°. Grease a 14-in. Pizza ; sprinkle with cornmeal. On a floured surface, roll dough into a 13-in. Circle.

2. Transfer to organized pan; increase edges slightly. Sprinkle with cheese, fowl and bacon. Bake till crust is gently browned 10-12 mins.

3. Meanwhile, vicinity romaine and arugula in a big bowl. In a small bowl, integrate mayonnaise, lemon juice, lemon zest, and pepper.

4. Pour over lettuces; toss to coat. Arrange overheat pizza. Top with tomato, avocado, and basil. Serve immediately.

Oriental Applebee Salad

Servings: 2 servings

Nutrition: Carbohydrates: 65g/ Protein: 60g/ Fat: 47g

Ingredients:

- 1 pound skinless chicken breast 2 portions
- 2 tablespoons olive oil
- 1/2 teaspoon salt
- 1/4 teaspoon black pepper
- 1/2 cup sliced almonds
- 8 cups romaine lettuce
- 1/4 cup shredded carrots
- 1/2 cup crispy rice noodles
- 4 tablespoons Applebees Oriental Salad Dressing

Instructions:

1. Heat the grill to medium, or warmness a solid iron skillet or grill pan over medium warmness. Place the hen breasts between two sheets of plastic wrap and lightly pound them to 3/8-inch thick.

Brush with the olive oil and season them with salt and pepper.

2. Grill for five to 7 minutes on each side, until cooked through.

Transfer to a plate to relaxation for four to 5 minutes earlier than slicing.

3. Toast the almonds in a small dry skillet over medium warmth

4. Oversee them—there's a high-quality line between toasted almonds and burnt almonds! Shake the pan gently. When you begin to odor the almonds, toast for some seconds more, then immediately area the almonds on a paper towel. Allow them to chill for a moment or.

5. Assemble salads by first putting down the lettuce, 3 to 4 cups consistent with serving.

6. Sprinkle every with 2 tablespoons of the carrots, 1/4 cup crispy rice noodles, and 1/four cup toasted almonds. Arrange the fowl on the pinnacle. Serve with masses of the Applebee's Oriental Salad Dressing.

Chick-fil-A Chicken Nuggets

Servings: 5 servings

Nutrition: Carbohydrates: 3g/ Protein: 19g/ Fat: 2g

Ingredients:

- 1 pound boneless, skinless chicken breasts
- 1/2 cup dill pickle juice
- 1/4 cup milk
- 2 teaspoons powdered sugar
- 1 1/2 teaspoons kosher salt
- 1 teaspoon black pepper
- 1/4 teaspoon garlic powder
- 1/4 teaspoon paprika
- 1/4 teaspoon celery salt
- 1/3 cup mayonnaise
- 1 tablespoon honey
- 2 teaspoons Dijon mustard
- 1 teaspoon yellow mustard
- 1 teaspoon apple cider vinegar
- 1/4 teaspoon kosher salt

Instructions:

1. Cut bird into bite-sized pieces—place in a bowl with pickle juice and milk. Marinate for 30 minutes. Remove from marinade and pat dry.

2. In a small bowl, combine powdered sugar, salt, pepper, garlic powder, paprika, and celery salt. Sprinkle all over the hen.

3. Heat grill to high. Grill hen for 3 minutes according to side till cooked through.

4. Serve with honey mustard dipping sauce.

Mexican pizza by Taco Bell

Servings: 4 servings

Nutrition: Carbohydrates: 34g/ Protein: 27g/ Fat: 24g

Ingredients:

- 1 pound ground beef
- 1 packet taco seasoning
- 3/4 cup water
- 1 cup vegetable oil
- 8 flour tortillas (taco size)
- 1 (15 oz) can refried beans
- 1 (10 oz) can enchilada sauce
- 2 cups shredded Mexican cheese blend
- diced tomatoes
- sliced green onion
- sliced olives
- sliced green onions

Instructions:

1. Preheat oven to 400f. In a big skillet, brown and crumble the ground beef.

2. Drain extra grease. Place cooked beef lower back in skillet and add taco seasoning packet and water and stir. Bring to a boil then lessen warmth and simmer till thickened.

3. In a considerable skillet, warmness up oil over medium warmness.

4. Add tortillas (one at a time) and cook dinner for 3-4 mins (flipping fre q uently) until crisp.

5. Continue with the rest of the tortillas. Set aside.

6. Meanwhile, warmness up the refried beans in a microwaveable-safe bowl. This will make it less complicated to unfold the beans onto the tortilla shells.

7. On each tortilla, slather a generous layer of refried beans. Then top with seasoned ground red meat.

8. Place every other tortilla on the pinnacle. Slather about tablespoons of the enchilada sauce on a pinnacle. Then location a few shredded kinds of cheese on top of the sauce. Continue assembling the rest of the pizzas.

9. Place the pizzas on a massive nonstick baking sheet and bake for approximately 8-10 minutes until cheese is melted. Serve along with your favorite toppings!

Steak n 'Shake Chili

Servings: 8 servings

Nutrition: Carbohydrates: 89g/ Protein: 49g/ Fat: 34g

Ingredients:

- 2 pounds ground chuck coarsely ground
- 1 1/2 cups onion diced
- 1 teaspoon celery salt
- 32 ounces tomato sauce
- 1 cup Water
- 28 ounces light kidney beans
- 2 teaspoons garlic powder
- 1 1/2 teaspoons garlic salt
- 2 tablespoons chili powder plus
- 1 teaspoon chili powder
- 1/2 teaspoon salt
- 1/2 teaspoon pepper
- 16 ounces tomato paste

Instructions:

1. Please note the onions which can be cooked inside the chili are optional. You can depart them out. I in my opinion, love onions while cooked in the chili.

2. Steak N Shake does now not upload onions to cooked chili.

Chopped onions are served on top of the chili.

3. In a skillet on medium-low warmness saute ground pork and onions. When the pork has been cooked, drain all grease and vicinity in a medium-huge saucepan. Add celery salt, tomato sauce, kidney beans, garlic powder, garlic salt, chili powder, pepper, water, and salt, mix all ingredients.

4. On low warmness place a lid on the saucepan and simmer for one hour, stirring frequently. After the chili has been cooking for an hour add tomato paste and stir well. Place lid at the pan and simmer a further half-hour. Prepare spaghetti as directed and drain.

5. To assemble: For person serving: In a shallow bowl or plate area: Generous helpings of spaghetti three/four cup Chili 2 tablespoon Chili Sauce Chopped Onions (to taste) 1/2 cup Shredded Monterey Jack and Colby Cheese Mix Top with extra onions for your taste.

Meatloaf of Cracker Barrel

Servings: 4 servings

Nutrition: Carbohydrates: 18g/ Protein: 31g/ Fat: 15g

Ingredients:

- 10 pounds ground beef
- 30 ounces of chopped onions, 1/4-inch pieces
- 1 pound green bell peppers, diced
- 10 eggs
- 5 tablespoons salt
- 1 1/2 tablespoons pepper
- 1 1/2 quart canned tomatoes, diced
- 2 1/4 cups biscuit crumbs, grated
- Catsup

Instructions

1. Preheat oven to 300 levels Fahrenheit.

2. Mix ground beef, onions, inexperienced bell peppers, eggs, salt, pepper, tomatoes, and biscuit crumbs completely with a gloved hand in a big bowl.

3. Divide into three loaf pans, pressing down with a spoon.

4. Using a convection oven, bake at 300 tiers Fahrenheit for 60 minutes.

5. Remove loaf pans from the oven.

6. Invert every loaf over an 8-inch wire rack to drain grease and juice.

7. Top every loaf with a half cup of catsup.

8. Slice into 5 to six-ounce quantities and preserve warm till equipped to serve.

DIY sparkling pan, Applebee cheese, and mushrooms

Servings: 4 -6 servings

Nutrition: Carbohydrates: 6g/ Protein: 4g/ Fat: 19g

Ingredients:

- l batch homemade pasta dough
- 1 tbsp olive oil
- oz (500g) Chestnut mushrooms (crimini) . sliced 2 shallots finely chopped
- 1 clove garlic
- 1 sprig thyme
- 1 heaped tbsp ricotta
- 2 tbsp parmesan freshly grated salt and pepper to season 1/2 tbsp olive oil
- 1 cup (250ml) double cream (heavy cream)
- 2 tbsp parmesan freshly grated
- 1 clove garlic
- 1 pinch nutmeg
- 1 sprig thyme salt and pepper
- 1 clove garlic
- 1 sprig thyme
- 1 heaped tbsp ricotta
- 2 tbsp parmesan freshly grated salt and pepper to season 1/2 tbsp olive oil
- 1 cup (250ml) double cream (heavy cream)
- 2 tbsp parmesan freshly grated
- 1 clove garlic
- 1 pinch nutmeg
- 1 sprig thyme salt and pepper

Instructions:

1. To Make The Filling

2. Heat a 1 tbsp of olive oil in a medium-sized pan, once warm upload the finely chopped shallots and saute till gentle and translucent.

3. Add the chopped mushrooms and cook down till contracted and softened. Add the garlic and thyme and a significant pinch of salt and pepper, fry for 1-2 minutes. Set apart and permit refreshing for 5 minutes.

4. Add the cooled mushroom combination to a food processor with Parmesan and ricotta. Blitz until clean and pate like.

5. To Make self-made egg pasta dough observe this recipe right here and comply with the method for rolling out. There are some vital tips you need.

6. Using homemade pasta dough, roll it out from the widest setting to the third closing setting. Lay one sheet of pasta down and the vicinity around 1 heaped tsp of mushroom aggregate inside the center of the pasta sheet 1 inch apart.

7. Fold one edge of the pasta over the filling to meet the alternative edge. You may need to softly pat the filling down at this point, so it folds simpler. Using your fingers seal the sides of the ravioli filling as shown.

8. Tip: Technically those are known as mezzaluna (half-moons) because they're folded over and don't have 4 sealed edges. These are slightly simpler to make for this reason, but in case you want to make conventional Ravioli indeed region the second sheet of pasta without delay on the pinnacle of the first and seal together with your arms.

9. Seal the top of the dough with your thumb while holding the two edges as shown in picture 10. This will make sure all of the air has escaped, which will forestall the ravioli bursting or going wrinkly.

10. Cut the Ravioli out both with a ravioli or pasta cutter, cookie cutter, or fluted pasta wheel and set apart on a surface sprinkled lightly with semolina or 00 flour even as you make the next batch.

11. Once the Ravioli (or mezzaluna) are geared up to deliver a massive pot of salted water to a boil. Add the Ravioli to the water and cook for round 4 mins. Meanwhile, make the sauce.

To Make The Sauce

Heat a little olive oil in a big pan and fry the chopped garlic for 1 minute.

Add the cream, thyme, nutmeg, salt and pepper. Stir and convey to a boil.

Let it boil for 30-forty seconds, then flip low and add the freshly grated Parmesan. Stir until slightly thickened flip off the warmth and upload the cooked Ravioli directly from the water the use of a slotted spoon.

Toss within the sauce and serve.

SOUP RECIPES

Creamy Tuscan soup from Copycat Olive Garden

Servings: 4 servings

Nutrition: Carbohydrates: 30g/ Protein: 17g/ Fat: 38g

Ingredients:

- 1 pound spicy Italian ground sausage use mild for kid-friendly
- 4 tablespoons butter
- 1/2 white onion, diced
- 1 tablespoon minced garlic
- 6 cups chicken broth
- 2 cups water
- 4/5 yellow potatoes, cut into 1-inch pieces
- 3 teaspoons salt or to taste
- 1 teaspoon black pepper
- 2 cups heavy cream
- 4 cups chopped kale
- chopped bacon or bacon bits and grated parmesan cheese for topping

Instructions:

1. In a large pot saute sausage 5-6 minutes till browned. Use a slotted spoon to transfer sausage to a plate and set aside.

2. In the same pot, add butter and saute onions over medium warmth until translucent. Add garlic and saute for another minute until fragrant.

3. Add chicken broth, water, potatoes, salt, and pepper and convey to a boil. Boil until potatoes are tender. Stir in kale, and heavy cream. Add sausage. Taste and upload salt and pepper if needed.

Serve garnished with grated parmesan cheese if desired.

Cheddar soup with Panera broccoli

Servings: 1 serve

Nutrition: Carbohydrates: 19.4g/ Protein: 21.8g/ Fat: 37.5g

Ingredients:

- 1 tablespoon butter
- ½ onion, chopped
- ¼ cup melted butter
- ¼ cup flour
- 2 cups milk
- 2 cups chicken stock
- 1 ½ cups coarsely chopped broccoli florets
- 1 cup matchstick-cut carrots
- 1 stalk celery, thinly sliced
- 2 ½ cups shredded sharp Cheddar cheese
- 1 pinch salt and ground black pepper to taste

Instructions:

1. Melt 1 tablespoon butter in a skillet over medium-high warmth.

Saute onion in warm butter till translucent, about 5 mins. Set aside.

2. Whisk 1/four cup melted butter and flour together in a big saucepan over medium-low warmness; cook until flour loses it's granular texture, including 1 to 2 tablespoons of milk if necessary to keep the flour from burning, 3 to four minutes.

3. Gradually pour milk into flour aggregate at the same time as whisking constantly. Stir chook inventory into milk combination. Bring to a simmer; prepare dinner until flour taste is long past and the combination is thickened, approximately 20 minutes. Add broccoli, carrots, sauteed onion, and celery; simmer till greens are tender, about 20 minutes.

4. Stir Cheddar cheese into vegetable aggregate till cheese melts.

Season with salt and pepper to flavor.

Inland baked potato soup

Servings: 8 servings

Nutrition: Carbohydrates: 31.4g/ Protein: 8.6g/ Fat: 8.3g

Ingredients:

- 12 slices bacon
- ⅔ cup margarine
- ⅔ cup all-purpose flour
- 7 cups milk
- 4 large baked potatoes, peeled and cubed
- 4 green onions, chopped
- 1 ¼ cups shredded Cheddar cheese
- 1 cup sour cream
- 1 teaspoon salt
- 1 teaspoon ground black pepper

Instructions:

1. Place bacon in a large, deep skillet. Cook over medium warmth until browned. Drain, crumble and set aside.

2. In a stockpot or Dutch oven, soften the margarine over medium warmness. Whisk in flour until smooth. Gradually stir in milk, whisking constantly until thickened. Stir in potatoes and onions.

Bring to a boil, stirring fre q uently.

3. Reduce warmness, and simmer 10 minutes. Mix in bacon, cheese, sour cream, salt, and pepper. Continue cooking, stirring fre q uently, until cheese is melted

Copycat Pasta and Beans from Olive Garden
Servings: 5 servings

Nutrition: Carbohydrates: 70g/ Protein: 35g/ Fat: 14g

Ingredients:

- 1 cup pasta, uncooked
- 1 pound Italian sausage
- 1 cup carrot, diced
- 1 cup celery, chopped
- 3/4 cup chopped yellow onion
- 1 clove minced garlic
- 3 (8-ounce) cans tomato sauce
- 3 cups beef broth
- 1 cup water
- 1 (15-ounce) can diced tomato, undrained
- 1 tablespoon plus 1 teaspoon granulated sugar
- 1 1/2 teaspoons dried basil
- 1 1/2 teaspoons dried thyme
- 1/2 teaspoon dried marjoram
- 1 (15-ounce) can dark red kidney beans, drained and rinsed 1 (15-ounce) can great northern beans, drained and rinsed salt and ground black pepper to taste

Instructions:

1. Cook sausage in skillet and set aside.

2. In Large stockpot sauté carrot, celery and onion the use of a touch olive oil, until onion is translucent and veggies are tender.

Add garlic and sauté for 45 seconds.

3. To this mixture, upload tomato sauce, broth, water, canned tomatoes, and all spices.

4. Salt and pepper to flavor (or wait and do this on end), changing heat to low.

5. Cover and prepare dinner at a simmer for a half-hour, stirring every 8 mins or so— Cook pasta.

6. Add cooked pasta to the soup in the stockpot, as well as the beans and allow to warm through.

7. Add extra broth as desired.

Carrabba minestrone

Servings: 1 yield bowl of soup

Nutrition: Carbohydrates: 51g/ Protein: 23g/ Fat: 9g

Ingredients:

- 2 teaspoons olive oil
- 1 large stalk celery diced small
- 2 large carrots sliced
- 1/2 small onion diced
- 4 cloves garlic minced
- 1/4 teaspoon salt or to taste
- 1/8 teaspoon black pepper or to taste
- 1/2 cup green beans snapped in 1 inch pieces 1 small yellow (summer) s q uash quartered and sliced 1 small zucchini squash quartered and sliced
- 4 cups green cabbage diced
- 1 tablespoon fresh parsley chopped
- 1/2 tablespoon basil (dried)
- 2 bay leaves
- 1 32-oz box vegetable broth low sodium, or low sodium chicken broth 4 cups water
- 1 14-oz can diced tomatoes
- 1.5 cups red potatoes diced
- 1 inch Parmesan cheese rind, or 2 T parmesan shavings 1 14-oz can garbanzo beans rinsed and drained
- 1 14-oz can cannellini beans (white kidney beans) rinsed and drained 1 14-oz can kidney beans rinsed and drained

Instructions:

1. Heat butter and oil and sauté celery, onion, carrots and garlic and cook dinner till soft.

2. Add green beans, cabbage, zucchini, parsley and basil and cook dinner until soft.

3. Add hen stock, bay leaf, tomatoes, prosciutto, romano rind and potatoes.

4. Allow soup to boil and immediately reduce to simmer. Simmer for 20-half-hour or until potatoes are soft. Add canned beans with their juices and simmer 5 mins more. Remove romano rind and prosciutto. Add grated romano cheese, stirring constantly.

Applebees tomato basil soup

Servings: 4 servings

Nutrition: Carbohydrates: 26g/ Protein: 5g/ Fat: 20g

Ingredients:

- 1 teaspoon Olive oil
- 1/2 cup Onion ; minced
- 2 28 ounce cans Crushed Tomatoes
- 2 cups V-8 Juice
- 1 cup Chicken broth
- 2 cloves Garlic ; minced
- 14 leaves Fresh basil; (Use up to 18 for stronger flavor) 1/2 teaspoon Italian Seasoning
- 1 1/4 cup Heavy cream
- Salt
- pepper

Instructions:

1. Heat 1 teaspoon olive oil in a huge saucepan and saute onion and garlic in olive oil.

2. Place tomatoes, juice and chicken broth/stock in a saucepan with onions and garlic, over medium heat; simmer 30 minutes. Puree the tomato aggregate alongside the basil leaves, onions, garlic and Italian Seasoning.

3. Turn heat to LOW heat. SLOWLY add heavy cream; season with salt and pepper as needed.

4. Simmer on low for 1? - 2 hours on low. Be sure the soup does now not boil.

Lemon Chicken Ozrp Soup

Servings: 6 bowls

Nutrition: Carbohydrates: 23.7g/ Protein: 23.9g/ Fat: 11.8g

Ingredients:

- 2 tablespoons olive oil, divided
- 1 pound boneless, skinless chicken thighs, cut into 1-inch chunks
- Kosher salt and freshly ground black pepper
- 3 cloves garlic, minced
- 1 onion, diced
- 3 carrots, peeled and diced
- 2 stalks celery, diced
- 1/2 teaspoon dried thyme
- 5 cups chicken stock
- 2 bay leaves
- 3/4 cup uncooked orzo pasta
- 1 sprig rosemary
- Juice of 1 lemon
- 2 tablespoons chopped fresh parsley leaves

Instructions:

1. Heat 1 tablespoon olive oil in a massive stockpot or Dutch oven over medium heat. Season chicken thighs with salt and pepper, to taste. Add chook to the stockpot and cook dinner until golden, approximately 2-three mins; set aside.

2. Add the remaining 1 tablespoon oil to the stockpot. Add garlic, onion, carrots and celery. Cook, occasionally stirring, till tender, approximately three-4 minutes. Stir in thyme until fragrant, about 1 minute.

3. Whisk in bird inventory, bay leaves and 1 cup water; bring to a boil. Stir in orzo, rosemary and chicken; reduce warmness and simmer until orzo is tender about 10-12 minutes.

4. Stir in lemon juice and parsley; season with salt and pepper, to taste serve immediately.

Thai Chicken Coconut Milk Soup

Ingredients:

- 1 lemongrass stalk - 6 cups chicken broth - 2 chicken breasts - 4 kaffir lime leaves
- 2 fresh and chopped red chili peppers
- 1 piece of ginger the size of a thumb and grated 400 ml of good quality coconut milk
- 2 tablespoons fish fumet (or more to taste)
- 2 tablespoons lemon juice - A handful of fresh basil leaves
- A handful of fresh coriander leaves
- OPTIONAL: Sliced pepper (or cherry tomatoes)
- OPTIONAL: 1 teaspoon brown sugar OPTIONAL: wheat or rice noodles

Direction:

1. Cut and chop the bottom of the lemongrass stalk. Keep the top stem for later.

2. Put the hen stock in a massive pot and produce to medium-high warmness. If you have leftover chook or turkey bones, upload them too.

3. Let it boil.

4. Add sliced skinless hen breasts and mushrooms.

5. Next, upload the lemongrass, the upper stem, the kaffir lime leaves, and the fresh chiles.

6. Boil for 5 to 8 minutes or until the fowl is cooked correctly. Lower the heat to medium.

7. Add ginger, two hundred ml of coconut milk, fish sauce, and additional veggies (if you use). Stir well and simmer for a couple of mins. Lower the warmth.

8. Add the lime juice and stir.

9. Do tastes test. Find the stability among acidic, spicy, salty, and candy flavors. Start with salinity; add greater fish fumet if the soup isn't salty or tasty enough, one tablespoon at a time. If it's miles very bitter, upload brown sugar. If the soup could be intensely spicy or in case you need it to be creamier, upload more fabulous coconut milk. If it isn't tasty enough, upload more chiles.

10. Serve Thai fowl soup in serving bowls. Sprinkle some fresh cilantro, chives, and basil over each bowl.

11. If you are going to serve the soup with noodles, it's far better to put together them separately; otherwise, the soup turns into thick because of the starch of the noodles.

Nutrition: Calories 357 Calories from Fat 63% Protein 29g Fat 25g Sat fat 19g Carbohydrate 7.2g Fiber 0.5g Sodium 484mg Cholesterol 79mg

Corn Cream Recipe

Ingredients:

- 1 ear of corn
- 1 yellow pepper
- 1 onion
- 1 tablespoon butter
- 1 splash of cream
- Vegetable soup
- 1 dash of extra virgin olive oil

Direction:

1. Place the butter in a pan and brown the formerly peeled and finely chopped onion.

2. When the onion is transparent, add the yellow pepper cut into small cubes along with the corn and a drizzle of more fabulous virgin olive oil.

3. When the greens are golden brown, cowl with the vegetable stock.

4. Crush the instruction with a touch of cream or milk cream and serve the new corn cream. Garnish with corn kernels and chopped parsley.

Nutrition: Per serving: 253 calories; 16.5 g fat; 24.8 g carbohydrates; 5.1 g protein; 54mg cholesterol; 373 mg sodium.

Zucchini cream

Ingredients:

- 3 medium zucchini
- 1 onion
- 1 large potato
- ½ leek
- 200ml of water
- 100ml of cream or liquid cream
- 30ml olive oil
- 1 tablet of chicken broth

Direction:

1. Wash all the vegetables.

2. Chop the zucchini, leek, onion, and potato into small cubes.

3. Heat the olive oil in a pot and sauté the onion and the leek. Add the zucchini and potato and sauté for 5 minutes or till the zucchini takes a bit color.

4. Add a tablet of broth and a tumbler of water and cook dinner for 20 higher mins.

5. Remove from warmth and mash the veggies with the blender until you get a creamy texture. Finally, add the cream and mix.

Season with salt and ground black pepper.

Pumpkin cream soup

Ingredients:

- 1 pumpkin of 1 kilo or pumpkin
- ¼ onion
- 2 butter spoons
- 2 tablespoons flour
- 2 tablespoons olive oil
- ¾ cups of cream or milk cream Toasted bread
- 2 cups chicken broth
- A handful of chopped fresh parsley Salt and ground black pepper

Direction:

1. Cut the squash into pieces and take away the seeds and fibers by using scraping with a spoon.

2. Place the pumpkin in a microwave-safe box and cook dinner for 10 mins. Remove, and if it is soft, take away the peel and region the pulp in a blender collectively with the hen broth. Blend until it's miles absolutely ground. If you do no longer have a microwave oven, do now not worry, because you can prepare dinner the pumpkin reduce into pieces in water until it's miles very tender or even make it baked.

3. Put the butter and oil in a pot and produce it to the fire when hot add the peeled and finely chopped onion and cook until transparent.

4. Add the flour and mix quickly. Cook for a few minutes until golden brown.

5. Pour the liquid pumpkin and prepare dinner over medium warmness for 10 minutes, stirring occasionally.

6. Season with salt and floor black pepper to taste and add the cream or milk cream. Cook for a couple of mins. If the pumpkin cream soup is very thick, you may add water or chicken broth.

7. Serve the pumpkin cream soup on a soup plate or in bowls and decorate with portions of toast, parsley, and pumpkin seeds.

Nutrition: Per Serving: 322 calories; 25.4 g fat; 20.2 g carbohydrates; 5.1 g protein; 83mg cholesterol; 1313 mg sodium.

Pumpkin cream with edible mushrooms

Ingredients:

- 1 large pumpkin
- 500c.c. chicken broth
- 350g edible mushrooms
- 100g grated Parmesan cheese
- 1 onion
- 2 cloves of garlic
- A splash of liquid cream
- Salt and nutmeg c / n
- Olive oil c / n

Direction:

Clean the pumpkin and peel it.

1. Cut it in 1/2 and skip a peeled garlic clove so that the pulp is impregnated with the flavor.

2. Place on a tray; pour a touch olive oil over the pumpkin and bake for 60 mins at 250 ° C.

3. After this era of time, an area the baked pumpkin in a saucepan with the bird stock and the peeled onion; cook for 20 mins.

4. When the squash is soft, crush everything in a blender.

5. Add some grated Parmesan cheese and maintain crushing.

6. Place a few olive oils with the last garlic clove peeled and chopped and sauté the rolled edible mushrooms. When the mushrooms are cooked, reserve them.

7. Serve the pumpkin cream in soup dishes or clay casseroles with a little grated Parmesan cheese, salt, and nutmeg, cream, and mushrooms.

FISH, BEEF AND CHICKEN RECIPES

Alice Springs chicken from the Outback

Servings: 7 servings

Nutrition: Carbohydrates: 9.4g/ Protein: 57.5g/ Fat: 37.7g

Ingredients:

- 0.88 cup Dijon mustard - 0.88 cup honey - 0.44 cup mayonnaise
- 1.75 teaspoon fresh lemon juice
- 7 boneless skinless chicken breast (about 1 1/2 pounds) tablespoons butter
- 14 ounces mushrooms sliced - 1.75 tablespoon olive oil
- 7 slices cooked bacon chopped into 2-inch pieces cups shredded Colby Jack cheese
- tablespoons fresh parsley for garnish, optional

Instructions:

1. In a small bowl, whisk collectively mustard, honey, mayonnaise, and lemon juice. Reserve ¼ cup sauce in a protected container and refrigerate till serving time.

2. Meanwhile, an area the hen breast in a big plastic zipper-top bag. Pour in the last sauce and flip in the bag till evenly coated. Refrigerate half-hour or overnight.

3. Next, preheat oven to 400 degrees. In a sizeable oven-evidence skillet over medium-high warmness, heat butter until the foaming.

4. Add mushrooms and sauté till they have launched most of their liquid and have commenced showing brown, about 5 to 7 mins.

5. Transfer to a bowl and wipe out skillet.

6. To the same skillet, heat oil till shimmering. Add hen (discarding any final marinade) in a single layer and do now not move until a golden-brown crust forms, approximately five mins. Flip each piece and retain to prepare dinner till the second side is browned, approximately 5 mins longer.

8. Divide the mushrooms frivolously over the fowl. Top with bacon and cheese. Cover the skillet and area in the oven. Bake until the hen reaches 165°F when examined with an internal thermometer on the thickest part, about 10 to 15 minutes.

9. Remove from oven and garnish with parsley if desired. Serve with reserved sauce on the facet for dipping.

Panda Express "Orange Chicken

Servings: 8 servings

Nutrition: Carbohydrates: 64g/ Protein: 33g/ Fat: 13g

Ingredients:

- 2 lb boneless, skinless chicken thighs (905 g) 1 tablespoon salt
- 1 teaspoon white pepper
- 1 cup cornstarch (125 g)
- 3 cups flour (375 g)
- 1 egg
- 1 ½ cups water (360 mL)
- 2 tablespoons oil
- 6 cups oil (1 ½ L), for frying
- 1 tablespoon oil
- ¼ teaspoon chili flake
- 1 tablespoon garlic, minced
- ½ teaspoon ginger, minced
- ¼ cup sugar (50 g)
- ¼ cup brown sugar (55 g)
- ¼ cup orange juice (60 mL)
- ¼ cup white distilled vinegar (60 mL)
- 2 tablespoons soy sauce
- 2 tablespoons water
- 2 tablespoons cornstarch
- 1 teaspoon sesame oil

Instructions:

1. On a cutting board, reduce bird into 1x1-inch (2x2-cm) cubes and set aside.

2. In a medium mixing bowl, combine salt, white pepper, cornstarch, and flour. Whisk to integrate.

3. Add the egg, water, and oil till it reaches the consistency of pancake batter.

4. Add the hen to the batter and refrigerate as a minimum of 30 minutes.

5. Heat oil in a wok or large backside pan to 350°F (180°C).

6. Gently add the hen and prepare dinner for 5-6 minutes till lightly golden brown.

7. Remove the bird from the pan and switch to a paper towel-coated plate.

8. Set a heavy-bottomed pot over medium-high warmness and upload the oil.

9. Once the oil starts to shimmer, upload the red pepper flakes, ginger, and garlic, and cook dinner for 30 seconds, stirring constantly.

10. Add the sugar and brown sugar, and stir to combine.

11. Add in the orange juice and permit the sugars to start to dissolve in the liquid, stirring occasionally.

12. Add within the vinegar and soy sauce, and stir to combine.

13. Add the cornstarch and water collectively and whisk to combine.

Add to the pan and stir.

14. Continue to prepare dinner the sauce till maple syrup consistency is achieved.

15. Add inside the fried bird and stir till completely coated within the sauce.

16. Top with sesame oil.

17. Enjoy!

Chili's Boneless Buffalo Wings

Servings: 2 servings

Nutrition: Carbohydrates: 28 g/ Protein: 23 g/ Fat: 47 g

Ingredients:

- 1 cup all-purpose flour - 2 tsp salt
- 1/4 tsp cayenne pepper - 1/2 tsp black pepper
- 1/4 tsp paprika
- 1 egg
- 1 cup milk
- 2 chicken breast fillets
- 1 vegetable oil for frying
- 1/4 cup Crystal or Frank's Louisiana hot sauce 1 tbsp margarine

Extra

- 1 celery
- 1 bleu cheese or ranch dip

Instructions:

1. Combine flour, salt, cayenne pepper, black pepper, and paprika in a medium bowl.

2. In every other small bowl whisk collectively egg and milk.

3. Slice every chicken breast into 6 portions.

4. Dip each piece of the bird into the egg mixture, then into the dry mix. Repeat so that each piece it's double-coated.

5. Chill for 15 minutes.

6. Heat vegetable oil (four-6 cups) to 375°F in a fryer or on the stove.

7. Drop bird in the oil and fry till each piece is browned. (Fry 2-3 pieces at a time)

8. Combine warm sauce and margarine in a small saucepan.

9. Heat over low warmth till margarine is melted.

10. Place chook in a container with a lid.

11. Pour sauce over the hen.

12. Cover and gently shake till chicken is coated correctly.

13. Serve on a plate with dip and celery.

Original fried chicken KFC Make-At-Home

Servings: 4-6 servings

Nutrition: Carbohydrates: 21.139g/ Protein: 53.20g/ Fat: 27.62g

Ingredients:

- Chicken drumsticks/breast
- Curd
- Egg (beaten),
- all-purpose flour
- bread crumbs
- chili powder
- white pepper powder
- onion (dried)
- basil/tulsi leaves (dried)
- oregano
- green chili
- garlic (dried), ginger (dried)
- salt
- Oil (for frying)

Instructions:

1. Wash and easy fowl. Drain water properly from the hen.

2. Add overwhelmed egg, curd, 1/2 tsp chili powder, salt to the chicken and blend nicely. Marinate it for a minimum of three to 4 hours.

3. Mix all reason flour, inexperienced chilies, white pepper, oregano, garlic, ginger, basil or tulsi leaves, closing chili powder, and salt.

4. Cover marinated chook with highly spiced all-cause flour blend and then with bread crumbs.

5. Heat oil in a thick bottom kadai and deep fry the chook in a gradual fire until it's miles cooked.

6. Serve hot with tomato ketchup.

Rotisserie Chicken Copycat at Boston Market

Servings: 4 servings

Nutrition: Carbohydrates: 8g/ Protein: 41g/ Fat: 12g

Ingredients:

- ¼ cup apple cider vinegar
- ½ cup canola oil
- 2 tablespoons brown sugar
- 4 fresh garlic cloves (minced)
- 1 whole roasting chicken

Instructions:

1. Mix all elements collectively and pour over fowl in a nonreactive bowl.

2. Let the chook marinate overnight.

3. In the morning, turn the hen to marinate the alternative side.

4. Several hours later, pull the chook out of the fridge and let it rest for 20 mins or when it has come to room temperature.

5. I in my view placed this in my infant George rotisserie oven but you may bake this on 350 for around 45 minutes to an hour or until the temperature within the thickest a part of the thigh has reached a hundred and sixty degrees.

Cracker Barrel Chicken and dumplings

Servings: 8 servings

Nutrition: Carbohydrates: 55g/ Protein: 37g/ Fat: 9g

Ingredients:

- 2 cups flour
- 1/2 teaspoon baking powder
- 1 pinch salt
- 2 tablespoons butter
- 1 cup milk
- 2 quarts chicken broth
- 3 cups cooked chicken

Instructions:

1. In a bowl, integrate the flour, baking powder, and salt. Cut the butter into the dry substances with a fork or pastry blender. Stir in the milk, mixing with a fork until the dough paperwork a ball.

2. Heavily flour a piece surface. You'll need a rolling pin and something to cut the dumplings with. I like to apply for a pizza cutter. I additionally like to use a small spatula to lift the dumplings off the cutting surface.

3. Roll the dough out skinny with a heavily floured rolling pin. Dip your cutter in flour and reduce the dumplings in squares approximately 2x2-inches every. It's okay for them now, not to be exact. Just eyeball it. Some can be bigger, a few smaller, and some might be formed funny.

4. Use the floured spatula to put them on a closely floured plate.

Just hold flouring between the layers of dumplings.

5. To cook dinner them, bring the broth to a boil. Drop the dumplings in one at a time, stirring at the same time as you upload them. The more flour on them will assist thicken the broth.

6. Cook them for approximately 15 to twenty minutes or until they don't flavor doughy.

7. Add the cooked hen to the pot and serve.

Copycat Wendy's Beef Chili

Servings: 10 servings

Nutrition: Carbohydrates: 6g/ Protein: 16g/ Fat: 18g

Ingredients:

- 2 pounds fresh ground beef
- 1 q uart tomato juice
- 1 (29-ounce) can tomato puree
- 1 (15-ounce) can red beans, drained
- 1 (15-ounce) can pinto beans, drained
- 1 large onion, chopped (about 1 1/2 cups)
- 1/2 cup diced celery
- 1/4 cup diced green bell pepper
- 1/4 cup chili powder
- 1 teaspoon cumin
- 1 1/2 teaspoons garlic powder
- 1 teaspoon salt
- 1/2 teaspoon ground black pepper
- 1/2 teaspoon oregano
- 1/2 teaspoon sugar
- 1/8 teaspoon cayenne pepper

Instructions:

1. In a skillet, brown the ground pork; drain.

2. Put the drained red meat and the remaining components in a 6-q uart pot.

3. Cover the pot; let it simmer for 1 to 1 1/2 hours, stirring every 15 minutes.

4. In a skillet, brown the ground beef; drain. Put the drained red meat and the last elements in a gradual cooker, turn on low and prepare dinner for four hours.

Salmon Gravlax

Ingredients:

2 salmon fillets of 1 kilo each, without skin

¼ cup vodka

1/3 cup fine sea salt

1/3 cup sugar

1 tablespoon ground black pepper

¼ cup chopped dill

Direction:

1. Gather the components of salmon gravlax.

2. Rinse the salmon fillets and dry them properly.

3. Use pliers or pliers to remove the spines if necessary.

4. Sprinkle the salmon flippantly with the vodka.

5. In a small bowl, combine sugar, pleasant sea salt, and floor black pepper.

6. Divide the aggregate into three identical parts within the bowl.

7. Put half of the one-0.33 of the curing aggregate on a rimmed baking sheet.

8. Place a skinless salmon fillet at the mixture and spread a third inside the aggregate at the fillet.

9. Spread the opposite 1/2 of the third over the second one steak and sprinkle each with chopped dill.

10. Place the second one fillet on the first and sprinkle the closing curing aggregate on the skin of the top salmon.

11. Cover the tray with foil and area a wood board on the blanketed fish. Cover with a heavy pot and produce it to the fridge for at least 12 hours.

12. Remove from the fridge and discard the gathered liquid inside the tray. Bring the salmon back in the refrigerator for 12 hours.

Its fish is already cured, and you could serve it. However, it'll continue to advantage of every other 12 to 24 hours of refrigeration.

Nutritional Guidelines (per serving):238 Calories 12g Fat 3g Carbs 27g Protein

Salmon with grilled eggplants and chickpea croutons

Ingredients:

- 3 tablespoon plus 1 teaspoon olive oil
- 1 onion, finely chopped
- 2 cloves garlic, minced
- 1 cup chickpea flour
- 1 tablespoon lemon zest2 teaspoons lemon juice 2 medium eggplants
- 600 g of skinless salmon fillet, cut into 4 pieces
- ¼ cup plain nonfat yogurt
- 1 cup mint leaves
- 2 tablespoons chopped chives

Direction:

1. Cover mildew with parchment paper.

2. Heat a tablespoon of oil in a pan and produce to medium warmness. Add one of the garlic and chopped onion and room to taste, constantly stirring, until the whole thing is tender, 3. Add two cups of water, and while it boils, upload the chickpea flour and beat vigorously, out of the warmness till there are nearly no lumps left.

4. Bring the aggregate to the lemon zest food processor and puree, step by step, including a tablespoon of oil till it is entirely smooth, Transfer to the mildew and cover with another piece of parchment paper. Put a mole up and press with a heavy object.

Refrigerate until firm.

5. Heat the grill to medium-high. Cut the chickpea combination into 1.5 cm cubes. Heat a teaspoon of oil in a small pan and cook dinner the chickpea croutons until golden brown, turning occasionally. Transfer to a paper towel to take away excess fat.

6. Slice the eggplant lengthwise and brush the eggplant slices with the relaxation of the oil. Sauté with salt and handle until gentle, 3 to 4 mins.

7. Season the salmon with salt and floor black pepper and add to the grill collectively with the eggplant and cook dinner for 5 minutes on each side.

8. In a small bowl, mix yogurt, chopped garlic clove, lemon juice, and salt. Sprinkle the yogurt sauce over the eggplants and accompany with chickpea croutons, chopped chives, and mint.

9. Serve with grilled salmon.

Zucchini noodles with shrimp

Ingredients:

- 750 g of peeled and deveined shrimp
- ¼ cup dry vermouth
- 1/3 cup lemon juice
- 5 zucchini
- 2 tablespoons unsalted butter
- 2 tablespoons chopped fresh parsley
- 2 tablespoons olive oil
- 2 tablespoons minced garlic
- 3 teaspoons lemon peel
- ½ teaspoon red pepper
- Parmesan cheese c / n
- Salt and ground black pepper to taste

Direction:

1. Create a zucchini zoodles with a spiralizer.

2. Season the shrimp with salt and floor black pepper.

3. Heat the butter and oil collectively in a pan over medium warmth. Once the butter melts, upload the garlic and shrimp.

4. Cook the shrimp for two to three minutes, till they are red and cooked. Remove and reserve.

5. Add the vermouth and lemon juice to the butter mixture and simmer for one or two mins.

6. Add the lemon zest, pink pepper, and chopped fresh parsley.

Add the zucchini and sauté for a further min till the zoodles are barely gentle and protected with the sauce.

7. Mix the shrimp with the noodles and serve with the grated Parmesan cheese.

Salmon piccata with lemon sauce

Ingredients:

- 4 skinless salmon fillets
- ½ teaspoon fat salt
- ½ teaspoon ground black pepper
- 3 tablespoons all-purpose flour
- 2 tablespoons olive oil
- 3 cloves garlic, minced
- ¼ cup dry white wine
- Juice of 2 lemons and slices to decorate
- 2 tablespoons capers
- 2 tablespoons chopped fresh parsley
- 2 teaspoons unsalted butter

Direction:

1. Gather all the elements of the salmon piccata.

2. Sprinkle the salmon and butter with flour. Shake the excess and cook the salmon fillets in a massive pan with warm oil for two mins, until they're browned on both sides.

3. Reduce heat to medium and add chopped garlic cloves; Continue cooking for a minute.

4. Add the drained lemon juice, wine, chopped sparkling parsley, and capers; Cook over medium-low warmness until the fish is nicely cooked, 5 to six minutes. Remove the pan from the warmth.

5. Add the butter; Stir until it melts, approximately 30 seconds.

6. Serve the salmon piccata with lemon sauce and enhance it with the slices.

Avocado and fish cake

Ingredients:

- Round puff pastry
- 3 avocados
- 125g smoked salmon
- 100ml evaporated milk
- Juice of half a lemon
- Get fat
- Garlic powder
- Fresh coriander
- Salt and ground black pepper

Direction:

1. Preheat the oven to 200 ° C.

2. Spread the puff pastry sheet on a tray greased with oil or butter and paint it with a beaten egg.

3. Place a sheet of aluminum foil over it and on this chickpeas or beans and bake for 12 mins or till golden brown. Let it cool. Peel avocados and remove the stone with a knife stroke. Remove the pulp with the help of a spoon and place it in a bowl with the evaporated milk and lemon juice.

4. Mix till a homogeneous preparation.

5. Add salt, garlic powder, and floor black pepper.

6. Spread the avocado cream over the puff pastry, as soon as cold.

Peel the last avocado and put off the corozo. Cut it into thin strips and placed them across the cake.

7. Crumble the smoked salmon and placed it in the center.

8. Finally, beautify the avocado and fish pie with fats salt and coriander leaves.

VEGETARIAN RECIPES

Applebee Low-Fat Quesadilla

Servings: 1 serve

Nutrition: Carbohydrates: 84g/ Protein: 48g/ Fat: 30g

Ingredients:

- ½ ounce shortening
- 2 (12 inch) flour tortillas
- 2 tablespoons chipotle hot sauce
- 4 ounces grilled chicken (Seasoning optional)
- 1 cup lettuce, shredded
- 4 ounces sour cream
- 2 ounces green onions
- 4 ounces salsa

Instructions:

1. Brush one facet of each tortilla with shortening.

2. Place one tortilla, shortening side down on the work floor.

Spread chipotle sauce evenly on one tortilla.

3. If hen was no longer freshly grilled, then microwave chicken approximately 45 seconds, then distribute calmly on the pinnacle of sauce on tortilla.

4. Evenly put Quesa Filling on top of fowl. Then, cowl with the other tortilla, shortening facet up.

5. Brown on griddle or in non stick pan frivolously on each side until inner filling is thoroughly heated.

6. Use shredded lettuce, sour cream, inexperienced onion, and salsa as accompaniments. I like to feature crumbled bacon on top.

DIY Quinoa California Salad From Whole Foods

Servings: 4 servings

Nutrition: Carbohydrates: 73g/ Protein: 14g/ Fat: 23g

Ingredients:

- 1/2 cup quinoa dry
- 1 cup water to cook quinoa
- 1 large mango chopped in small pieces
- 1/4 small red onion chopped
- 1/2 red bell pepper chopped
- 3/4 cup shredded coconut unsweetened
- 3/4 cup almond slices or slivers, toasted if preferred 1 cup raisins
- 1 cup edamame shelled, thawed if frozen 1/4 cup cilantro chopped, or parsley if you don't like cilantro

Instructions:

1. Cook the quinoa in line with package instructions. Let cool.

2. Whisk all the dressing ingredients together in a small bowl.

3. In a large bowl, toss all of the salad ingredients collectively along with the cooled quinoa and upload the dressing. Toss it nicely and serve cold.

Boston Market Pumpkin Casserole

Servings: 12 servings

Nutrition: Carbohydrates: 78g/ Protein: 5g/ Fat: 14g

Ingredients:

- 5 pounds sweet potatoes - 4 tablespoons butter
- 2 eggs slightly beaten - 1 teaspoon salt
- 1 teaspoon ground cinnamon
- 1/2 teaspoon vanilla extract
- 1/2 teaspoon ground nutmeg
- 1/2 cup dark brown sugar
- 1/4 cup heavy cream - Nonstick cooking spray
- 1/2 cup all-purpose flour
- 1 cup dark brown sugar
- 1/4 teaspoon salt - 1 cup quick-cooking oats
- 1/2 teaspoon ground cinnamon
- 1/4 pound butter - 2 cups miniature marshmallows

Instructions:

1. Preheat the oven to 350 stages F.

2. Wrap sweet potatoes in foil, region them on a baking sheet and bake for about 1 hour. After 1 hour, check using piercing with a fork; if you may pierce them quickly, they're finished baking. If no longer, bake them a little longer and check again. Allow the sweet potatoes to cool till you may cope with them, put off foil, and get rid of skins by way of actually pushing off the surfaces from the flesh of the potato.

3. Place the cooked potatoes right into a big bowl. If using canned sweet potatoes, skip the baking. Just open the cans and drain off the syrup. Mash the candy potatoes with the butter the usage of a pastry blender or a potato masher until mostly clean.

4. Add the eggs, salt, cinnamon, vanilla, and nutmeg and beat till you've got a uniform mixture. Add the brown sugar and cream and blend properly.

5. Combine the flour, brown sugar, salt, oats, and cinnamon in a medium bowl and stir together properly. Stir inside the 1/four pound butter with a fork till you have a crumbly mixture. If you had turned off the oven, heat it once more to 350 levels F. Lightly coat a nine x 13-inch baking pan with cooking spray.

6. I am spreading the candy potatoes inside the pan. Top with the marshmallows, then fall apart the oatmeal crust on the pinnacle of the marshmallows—Bake 30 to forty-five minutes.

DIY Sweet Potato Casserole from Ruth's Chris

Servings: 6 serves

Nutrition: Carbohydrates:/ Protein:/ Fat:

Ingredients:

- 1 cup brown sugar
- 1/3 cup flour
- 1 cup chopped nuts (pecans preferred)
- 1/3 stick butter -- melted (Do not omit or reduce this amount) 3 cups mashed sweet potatoes (Garnets looks best and I bake mine first)
- 1 cup sugar
- 1/2 teaspoon salt
- 1 teaspoon vanilla
- 2 eggs -- well beaten
- 1 stick butter -- (1/2 cup) melted (You can leave it out or reduce it, if you wish)

Instructions:

1. Combine brown sugar, flour, nuts and butter in mixing bowl. Set aside.

2. Preheat oven to 350 degrees.

3. Combine candy potatoes, sugar, salt, vanilla, eggs and butter in a mixing bowl within the order listed. Mix very well.

4. Pour the combination into a buttered baking dish.

5. Sprinkle the floor of the sweet potato aggregate evenly with the crust mixture.

6. Bake for 30 minutes. Allow setting at least 30 minutes before serving.

Olive Garden salad and creamy dressing

Servings: 12 servings

Nutrition: Carbohydrates: 8.9g/ Protein: 1.1g/ Fat: 10.2g

Ingredients:

- 1 packet Good Seasonings Italian Dressing
- Ingredients needed to make dressing; oil, water & vinegar
- ½ tsp dried Italian Seasoning ½ tsp table salt
- ¼ tsp black pepper
- ½ tsp sugar
- ¼ tsp garlic powder
- ½ tbsp mayonnaise
- ¼ cup olive oil
- 2 tbsp white vinegar
- 1 ½ tbsp water

Instructions:

1. Prepare Good Seasonings Italian Seasonings Dressing because it states on the back of the package (blending with oil, water & vinegar in the measurements given on packet)

2. Once prepared to pour it in a medium bowl, then add additional substances indexed above (beginning with dried Italian Seasoning).

3. Using a whisk, blend all elements till mixed very well combined.

4. Serve with your preferred salad fixings.

Chipotle's Copycat Corantro Lime Rice
Servings: 6 servings

Nutrition: Carbohydrates: 25g/ Protein: 3g/ Fat: 0g

Ingredients:

- 1 cup uncooked basmati rice
- 2 cups reduced-sodium chicken broth
- 1/4 teaspoon kosher salt
- 1/8 teaspoon ground nutmeg
- 2 tablespoons lime juice
- 2 tablespoons minced fresh cilantro

Instructions:

1. Rinse the rice nicely under cold, walking water until it runs clear. This eliminates the excess starch molecules from the outside of the rice.

2. Place the rice, bird broth, and salt in a small saucepan. Bring the combination as much as a boil over medium-excessive warmth 3. Reduce the heat to low and cook dinner, covered, for 12 to 15 minutes, till the rice has absorbed all the liquid.

4. Allow the rice to sit, undisturbed, for 10 minutes before stirring.

5. Once the rice has rested, add the nutmeg, lime juice, and fresh cilantro. Fluff the mixture with a fork.

6. Serve immediately.

Copy Jalapeño-Cilantro Hummus by Panera

Servings: 2 servings

Nutrition: Carbohydrates: 12g/ Protein: 29g/ Fat: 35g

Ingredients:

- 6 cups spinach leaves
- 1 tomatoes Large, sliced
- 1/2 cucumber a Large, sliced
- 1/2 purple onion a Small, sliced
- 2 chicken breasts
- hummus Jalapeno Lime

Instructions:

1. For the hummus, combine all hummus ingredients in a meals processor and puree till smooth. Transfer mixture to a storage box and refrigerate till needed.

2. Combine paprika and fowl seasoning and set aside. To make hen, pound bird breasts to an even thickness. Season both facets with salt and pepper and paprika and fowl seasoning.

3. Heat oil in a large nonstick skillet to medium heat. Add bird breasts and cook 10-12 minutes or until done. Remove to a plate to permit refreshing. Then thinly slice.

4. Place ~2 to three cups of spinach in a massive salad bowl.

Decoratively top with tomatoes, cucumbers, purple onions, grilled hen slices (~half huge fowl breast in line with salad), a 1/2 of a lemon, and a scoop of cilantro-jalapeno hummus and a hearty sprinkle of chopped cilantro.

5. Enjoy!

Copycat Cici's Spinach-Alfredo Pizza

Servings: 8 slices

Nutrition: Carbohydrates: 22.1g/ Protein: 13.5g/ Fat: 19g

Ingredients:

- 1 cup classico alfredo sauce
- 25 leaves spinach
- ¼ cup mozzarella cheese, shredded
- ¼ cup parmesan cheese, shredded
- pizza dough (enough for one 12-inch pizza)

Instructions:

1. Roll out the fresh pizza dough right into a 12 inch circle, and region onto your stone or sheet.

2. Spread the alfredo sauce around and out to the edges and then lay the spinach on top of that, making sure not to overlap portions of spinach.

3. Then sprinkle cheeses on top and bake at 475 for 10-13 mins, or whatever you generally bake your pizza pie at.

Burger & Sandwich Copycat recipes

Servings: 6 burgers

Nutrition: Carbohydrates: 14.4g/ Protein: 19.9g/ Fat: 8g

Ingredients:

- Olive oil cooking spray
- 1 pound lean or very lean ground beef
- 1 cup shredded lettuce
- 1/4 cup onion minced
- 3 slices of Cheddar cheese
- 6 slider buns - 1/2 cup light mayo
- 1.5 Tablespoons ketchup
- 1 Tablespoon sweet relish
- 1 tsp dill pickle juice
- 1 Tablespoon minced onion
- 1/8 teaspoon garlic powder
- 1/8 teaspoon paprika
- 1/8 teaspoon onion powder
- 1/8 teaspoon ground mustard

Instructions:

1. Preheat oven to 350 levels F.

2. Spray the bottom of a 13x9 inch baking pan with olive oil spray.

3. Spread out the ground beef flippantly on the bottom of the organized baking pan.

4. Bake ground pork inside the oven for 20 minutes or until the temperature is 160 tiers F.

5. While beef is cooking, prepare the sauce: location all components in a small bowl and blend until combined.

6. When beef is cooked eliminated from the pan and cut into 12 same squares.

7. Place lettuce on the lowest of a slider bun.

8. Top with one beef patty.

9. Next, add cheese (half of one slice is good).

10. Top cheese with every other patty and then pickles.

11. Spread sauce on the pinnacle of the slider bun and add a pinch of onion.

Sonic's Signature House Burger

Servings: 6 servings

Nutrition: Carbohydrates: 10g/ Protein: 24g/ Fat: 50g

Ingredients:

- 1 1/2 cups Tater Tots
- 1 pound ground sausage
- 1/2 pound bacon
- 6 ounces American cheese
- 4 tablespoons milk, divided use
- 10 Eggs - salt and pepper
- 1/2 cup shredded Cheddar cheese
- 1 jalapeno pepper slices
- 6 flour tortillas

Instructions:

1. Preheat the oven to 350 degrees. Spray a baking sheet with nonstick spray and area the Tater Tots at the baking sheet.

2. Bake for approximately 22 to 25 mins. While the tater children are inside the oven, cook the sausage in a skillet over medium warmth till it is properly browned. Drain sausage over paper towels and cowl with some other paper towel to help hold the warmth in as you still prepare dinner the breakfast.

4. You can prepare dinner the bacon in the same pan that you cooked the sausage in. Cook the bacon until crispy.

5. Remove bacon from pan and drain on paper towels. Sonic serves their burrito with a cheese sauce.

6. Cube the 6 oz of American cheese and location in a small pot over low warmness and upload 2 tablespoons of milk. Melt the cheese, stirring frequently, the milk and cheese will combine to shape a cheese sauce.

7. Once the cheese sauce has fashioned flip off the burner and go away the pot at the stovetop, the residual heat will preserve the sauce fluid at the same time as you cook the eggs.

8. In a medium-sized bowl integrate the eggs with the ultimate 2 tablespoons of milk. Spray a nonstick skillet with nonstick spray. Over medium heat add the egg and milk combination.

9. Season eggs with a pinch of salt, and a pinch of black pepper.

Gently stir the eggs as they cook. Once they are done get rid of from the warmth.

10. Heat tortillas for about 60 seconds to make them heat and pliable eggs as they cook. Once they are done, get rid of the warmth.

11. Heat tortillas for about 60 seconds to make them heat and pliable.

12. Assemble these with the aid of distributing the eggs, sausage, tater tots, bacon, and cheese sauce over the tortillas.

13. If you need to upload a few jalapeno slices to the burritos do so, if you desire, add a little sprinkle of Cheddar cheese earlier than folding the burritos. If desired you could fold up the burritos, and wrap in plastic, and region inside the freezer so you can reheat later.

DIPS AND SAUCES

Copycat Friendly's Peanut Sauce

Ingredients:

- ¾ cup unsweetened peanut butter (look at the parts, many brands have sugar)
- 1 cup of milk
- 2 tablespoons oil or butter
- ½ cup finely chopped white onion
- 1 teaspoon ground cumin
- 1 teaspoon ground achiote
- 1 tablespoon finely chopped cilantro
- 3 tablespoons white onion, thinly sliced
- 1 hard-boiled egg, finely chopped (optional)
- 1 chili pepper, minced (optional and to taste) Salt to taste

Preparation:

1. Dissolve peanut butter with ½ cup of milk.

2. Heat the oil or butter to put together a refrito with the onion, achiote, cumin, and salt; prepare dinner until the onions are soft.

3. Add the dissolved peanut butter and the rest of the milk.

4. Mix well and simmer for 10 mins.

5. Add the chopped hard-boiled egg, chili pepper, cilantro, and chopped white onion. Serve the recent sauce.

Roasted tomato sauce

Ingredients:

- 1 1/2 kilos of tomatoes
- 3 tablespoon extra virgin olive oil
- 6 peeled garlic cloves
- 1/2 cup sliced onion
- 2 teaspoons Italian seasoning
- 1 teaspoon kosher salt
- 1/4 teaspoon freshly ground black pepper
- 3 tablespoons chopped basil
- Optional: 2 tablespoons tomato paste
- Optional: 500 g of pasta
- Optional: 1/8 teaspoon chopped red pepper flakes

Direction:

1. Gather the ingredients of the roasted tomato sauce and preheat the oven to a hundred and fifty °C.

2. Wash the tomatoes, cast off the stem, and reduce them into pieces of approximately 2 centimeters.

3. Mix the tomatoes in a massive bowl with olive oil, sliced onion, rolled garlic cloves, Italian seasoning, salt, and floor black pepper.

4. Place the tomatoes in a single layer on a baking sheet and bake for 60 mins.

5. Put roasted tomatoes and condiments in a meals processor or blender.

6. Mix properly and switch to a heavy saucepan and upload chopped basil, pink peppers, and tomato paste, in case you use them. Bring the roasted tomato sauce over low heat, and cook dinner for 15 mins or till reduced and thickened.

7. Cook the pasta in boiling water with salt; drains Mix the drained hot pasta with the sauce and serve with garlic bread in case you wish.

8. If you aren't going to apply the sauce immediately, region it in a box or glass jars with a lid and refrigerate and eat for up to a few days or store it within the freezer for up to four months.

Chick Fil A Sauce (copycat)

Ingredients:

- 1/4 cup honey
- 2 tablespoons of yellow mustard
- 1/4 cup barbecue sauce I use Sweet Baby Rays
- 1 tablespoon of lemon juice
- 1 tablespoon of Dijon mustard
- 1/2 cup mayonnaise

Direction:

1. Note: Click on the times in the commands to start a kitchen clock while cooking.

2. Mix all the elements in a bowl and relax for 30 minutes to bring the flavors together.

3. If your sauce has no smoke (in case your BBQ sauce is sweeter than smoky), take a sprint of liquid smoke.

Nutrition: Calories: 147kcal Carbohydrates: 20 g Protein: 0 g Fat: 0 g Saturated fat: 0 g Cholesterol: 0 mg Sodium: 11 mg Potassium: 162 mg Fiber: 0 g Sugar: 16 g Vitamin C: 37,4 mg Calcium: 14 mg Iron: 1 mg

Ragù (Italian meat sauce)

Ragù is the classic Italian meat sauce, and although there are different versions, the one I will teach you next has a Tuscan style. As with most Italian sauces, start with a celery, carrot, and onion sauce that is chopped and roasted in olive oil. This is the same as with French Mirepoix.

Ingredients:

For the sofrito:

- 2 tablespoons olive oil - 1 cup chopped onion
- 1/2 cup chopped carrot
- 1/2 cup celery cut into small cubes For the ragù: 30 g dried porcini mushrooms
- 2 tablespoons tomato paste - 5 thin slices of prosciutto
- 120 g minced pork - 120 g ground beef
- 1/2 cup dry red wine - 350 g of tomato puree

Fine sea salt

- Freshly ground black pepper to taste
- Pinch of freshly grated nutmeg
- 1/2 teaspoon finely grated lemon zest

Direction

1. Gather the stir-fried elements. Heat the olive oil in a saucepan over medium-low warmth. Sauté the carrot, onion, and celery till they soften and decrease a little, and the onions are caramelized.

3. Gather the ingredients of the ragù.

4. Put the dried porcini mushrooms in a small bowl and cowl with heat water. Let stand for 15 minutes.

5. When the mushrooms soften, drain and store the water in a separate box. Chop the mushrooms finely and reserve.

6. Add the tomato paste to the sauce and cook dinner until it thickens.

7. Add floor pork and minced meat. Increase heat to brown and stir with a wooden spoon constantly. Add the wine and mix until it evaporates.

9. Add the chopped porcini and tomato puree. Stir and season with nutmeg, salt, and freshly ground black pepper.

10. Pour the mushrooms soaking water and if you have finished the ragù sauce, take it away from the warmth and upload the sofrito and the finely grated lemon zest.

McDonald's Tartar Sauce - copycat recipe

Ingredients:

- 1/2 cup mayonnaise
- Chopped 1 1/2 tablespoons of white onions
- 1 tablespoon of carrot finely diced 1 tablespoon of cucumber relish Do not use dill relish 1 1/2 teaspoon of sugar
- 1/4 teaspoon of salt

Direction:

Mix all the ingredients in a small bowl. It is best to shop this sauce in the refrigerator for about half-hour earlier than serving. You can maintain this inside the fridge for 7 days.

Nutrition: Calories: 135kcal Carbohydrates: 2 g Protein: 0 g Fat: 13 g Saturated fat: 2 g Sodium: 244 mg Sodium: 8 mg Fiber: 0 g Sugar: 1 g Vitamin A: 430IU Vitamin C: 0.3 mg Iron: 0.1 mg

Pesto sauce with nuts

Pesto is a sauce originally from the city of Liguria, Italy, whose main ingredient is basil. In addition to this ingredient, others such as garlic, pine nuts, olive oil, and Parmesan or pecorino cheese are added. The term pesto comes from the Genoese pestare, which means to crush or grind in a mortar, which is how sauce is traditionally prepared. There are many variants, and the one that I will teach you to make today is one of them that is equipped with basil, peppermint, and nuts.

Ingredients:

- 2 bunches of basil
- Several peppermint leaves
- One garlic clove
- 40 g of walnuts
- 40 g of pistachios
- 80 g hazelnuts
- 60 g grated Parmesan cheese
- Extra virgin olive oil Salt

Direction:

1. Wash the basil and peppermint leaves and dry them with paper napkins.

2. Peel the garlic clove and cut it in half, eliminates the germ, that's the bud that is inside.

3. Cut the garlic clove into portions and location it in a bowl along with the mint and basil leaves. Go crushing with mortar even as adding pistachios, nuts, hazelnuts, grated Parmesan cheese, a pinch of salt, and a dash of olive oil.

4. Although this can additionally be accomplished with the assist of a blender or meals processor, the key is to make the pesto delicious and have an excellent texture that is only carried out with the mortar.

5. Once you have equipped your pesto with nuts, reserve it in a tightly closed container till it is time to apply it.

Chocolate syrup

Ingredients:

- 1 1/2 cups of water
- 1 1/2 cups white sugar
- 1 cup of cocoa powder
- 1 pinch of salt
- 1 teaspoon vanilla extract

Direction:

Put water, sugar, cocoa, and salt in a saucepan. Heat over low warmness, continually stirring, till the aggregate thickens and starts offevolved to bubble.

Remove from warmness and add vanilla.

Serve this warm syrup on ice, cakes, or fruit.

Sweet and sour sauce

The sweet and sour sauce is a perfect sauce to change the flavor of any dish that requires it and is also very useful for dips such as chicken nuggets. It is also so soft and exquisite that you can use it to accompany meats, chicken, spring rolls, Asian dishes, and so on. It is super simple to make, and you will have it ready in just 5 minutes. Let's point the ingredients!

Ingredients:

- 3 tablespoons white vinegar
- 1 cup of orange juice
- 6 tablespoons sugar
- 1½ teaspoons soy sauce
- 4 drops of tabasco sauce
- ¼ teaspoon salt
- 4 tablespoons ketchup
- 1½ tablespoons cornstarch
- 2 tablespoons cold water

Direction:

1. Dissolve the cornstarch in water; set aside.

2. Pour the white or alcohol vinegar, orange juice, soy sauce, ketchup, and salt right into a saucepan and warmth over medium-high heat till the sugar dissolves completely.

3. Reduce the heat and contain the corn starch dissolved inside the water. Stir until it boils, and the education is transparent.

4. When the bittersweet sauce has thickened, cast off from heat and let cool before serving.

Cheese sauce recipe

The 4 cheese sauce is a variety of pasta sauces very delicious and easy to prepare since it is made from the white sauce, also known as béchamel sauce, and also has a fusion of four kinds of cheese: Roquefort or blue, mozzarella, Sardo and provolone, or others. This sauce is creamy and, apparently, it is an adaptation of a French sauce known as Mornay sauce. Let's go for the recipe!

Ingredients:

- 200 cc of cream or milk 80g provolone cheese
- 80g of Sardinian cheese
- 80g mozzarella cheese
- 30g blue cheese
- 500 cc of milk
- 45g butter
- 45g flour
- 1 clove garlic
- Thyme c / n
- Salt and ground black pepper c / n Nutmeg c / n

Direction:

1. To make the sauce four varieties of cheese, vicinity the butter in a pot and produce it to the hearth.

2. Let soften and upload the flour. Stir at once with a twine whisk to make a roux and cook dinner the pasta over the fireplace for some seconds. Place the milk in a saucepan collectively with a clove of peeled and crushed garlic and a little thyme. When it starts offevolved to boil, take away from warmness and permit stand protected for 15 mins.

3. Remove the thyme and garlic clove and warm the milk again.

Put it within the other pot and mix thoroughly with some rods.

Pepper to taste and add a little nutmeg. Cook for 2 mins as soon as it boils.

4. Add mozzarella, provolone cheese, Sardinian cheese or a few form of cheese with holes, and blue cheese. Bring the pot to the fireplace and mix with a timber spoon so that the cheeses melt.

5. Add cream or milk cream and reserve the sauce 4 styles of cheese.

Copycat Chipotle Mexican Grill Spicy Corn Salsa

Ingredients:

- 2 cups of frozen corn
- 1/4 cup of chopped coriander
- 2 teaspoons of finely chopped jalapeno seeds removed 1/4 cup of chopped roasted poblano pepper
- 2 teaspoons of chopped red onions
- 1/2 teaspoon of kosher salt
- 1 teaspoon of lime juice
- 1 teaspoon of lemon juice

Direction:

1. Allow frozen corn to thaw completely.

2. Preheat the oven to 425 degrees. Stir in Poblano pepper with vegetable oil. When the oven is hot, fry the pepper on each side for 6 to 8 mins. Take the pepper out of the oven. Let it settle down a bit, put off the tough skin.

3. Chopped jalapeno very fine. If you don't like heat, take away seeds earlier than chopping. You can also begin with 1 teaspoon of jalapeno more first than adding the second one teaspoon.

Finely chop the Poblano pepper.

4. Add chopped coriander, salt, bell pepper, and purple onions. Mix inside the lemon juice and lime juice. Mix the salsa well. Place inside the refrigerator for some hours before serving. This allows the flavors to marry together.

Nutrition: Calories: 34kcal Carbohydrate: 8 g Protein: 1 g Saturated fat: 1 g Sodium: 118 mg Potassium: 104 mg Fiber: 1 g Sugar: 1 g Vitamin A: 52IU Vitamin C: 7 mg Calcium: 1 mg Iron: 1 mg

Tzatziki sauce

Ingredients:

- 2 natural yogurts
- 1 cucumber
- 1 clove garlic
- 4 fresh mint leaves
- 1 teaspoon dill
- Lemon juice c / n
- Salt and ground black pepper c / n

Direction:

1. To make the Greek cucumber and yogurt sauce, peel the cucumber and open it in half.

2. Remove the seeds, grate it and allow it to drain in a colander with a little salt to dispose of extra water. Squeeze on occasion with a spoon to hurry up this process.

3. Dry between absorbent paper and positioned it in a bowl. Drain the yogurts in a colander and upload it to the pan.

4. Add the peeled and overwhelmed garlic clove, dill, chopped peppermint leaves, salt, floor black pepper to taste, and some drops of lemon juice.

5. Mix the ingredients thoroughly to obtain a tzatziki sauce, test, and rectify if necessary. Let stand in the refrigerator for 30 minutes and serve cold with veggies or portions of bread to spread or accompany beef, poultry, or fish.

Coffee and chocolate syrup recipe for ice cream, desserts, and milkshakes

Ingredients:

- For coffee syrup
- 200 ml of water
- 200 g of sugar
- 2 tablespoons instant coffee with or without caffeine For the chocolate syrup
- 120g bitter cocoa powder
- 225 g of sugar
- 240 ml of cold water
- 1/2 teaspoon salt
- 1 tablespoon vanilla extract

Direction:

1. Preparation of coffee syrup step by step

2. To make the coffee syrup, you'll must location the sugar in a saucepan at the side of the water and the tablespoons of instant espresso with or without caffeine.

3. Bring the medium-excessive temperature to the hearth and while it boils, decrease the heat to medium and allow it to boil for 3 minutes. Let cool to room temperature and then the area in a pitcher jar and hold inside the fridge for 4 weeks. If you need to prepare the slightly thicker espresso syrup, you may let it boil for a couple more minutes, or upload four extra tablespoons of sugar in step one.

4. Preparation of chocolate syrup step by way of step

5. To make the chocolate syrup, location the bitter cocoa powder in a case in conjunction with the salt and sugar. Mix with a spoon and upload the bloodless water.

6. Bring the chocolate syrup to medium warmth, and while it boils, stir nonstop for 3 minutes.

7. Remove from warmth and add vanilla extract. Let cool to room temperature and then go to a tumbler jar and hold inside the fridge for a month. Remember that the chocolate syrup will thicken while it's miles bloodless.

Homemade Pesto

Ingredients:

- 100 gr of basil leaves
- 200 gr of Parmesan cheese
- 75 gr of pine nuts
- 2 cloves of garlic
- 160 ml olive oil Salt

Direction:

1. We prepare the main factor of this self-made pesto recipe, basil.

You should separate the leaves of the stem well. This step is essential because the stem tends to bitter the flavor of the dish barely.

2. Next, we will wash and dry the basil thoroughly. We can position it on absorbent paper so that it leaves all of the water which can have fallen. Otherwise, if any trace remains, it can purpose it to rust and change the coloration and taste of the dish.

It will darken rapidly and prevent having that severe green color so characteristic.

3. Peel the garlic cloves and reduce them into small portions. We start to put together the pine nuts in a pan, sauté them without oil to gather that extraordinary roasted flavor.

4. In the blender glass, we can locate the cloves of garlic, pine nuts, basil, and cheese, with a little olive oil. We overwhelm it very well and start creating the most traditional pesto. The texture and taste are unmistakable. Prepare self-made pasta and revel in an, in reality, exquisite dish.

Nutrition: Calories: 407kcal Carbohydrates: 3 g Protein: 7 g Fat: 42 g Saturated fat: 25g Sodium: 773 mg Potassium: 143 mg Fiber: 0 g Sugar: 0 g Vitamin A: 425IU Vitamin C: 1.8 mg Calcium: 156 mg Iron: 1.2 mg

Hollandaise sauce

Ingredient:

- 200 gr. of butter 4 egg yolks
- juice of 1/2 lemon or 1 tablespoon of white wine a pinch of salt

Preparation of hollandaise sauce:

1. Melt the butter in a saucepan using putting off the foam that appears at the surface, and permit it temper.

2. Put the egg yolks in a bowl and beat them with a rod blender.

When they begin to assemble, add the melted butter little by using little, being careful now not to feature the serum. This is left in the bottom, even as stirring until you get a great cream.

3. Add the juice of 1/2 lemon or a tablespoon of white wine and a pinch of salt at the same time as stirring. Serve the hollandaise sauce.

Nutrition: Calories: 247kcal Carbohydrates: 0 g Protein: 2 g Fat: 26 g Saturated fat: 15g Sodium: 207 mg Sodium: 14 mg Sugar: 0 g Vitamin A: 905IU Vitamin C: 1.5 mg Calcium: 24 mg Iron: 0.4 mg

Red pesto

Ingredients:

- 50g grated Parmesan cheese
- 100c.c. Of olive oil
- 10 dried tomatoes
- 10 fresh basil leaves
- 1 tablespoon pine nuts
- 1 clove garlic

Direction:

1. Place the dried tomatoes in a bowl and allow them to soak for at least 20 minutes: drain and reserve.

2. Put a pan on the hearth without oil or butter and location them, stir once in a while so that they do not burn.

3. Place the dried tomatoes within the blender glass and add the roasted

4. pine nuts washed basil leaves, peeled and chopped garlic clove, grated Parmesan cheese, and olive oil.

5. Crush all of the ingredients until you get a thick crimson pesto sauce. Store the red pesto in a formerly sterilized glass jar. Close it thoroughly and maintain it inside the fridge for as much as 7 days.

Carrot mayonnaise

Ingredients:

- 3 carrots
- ½ cup olive oil
- Fresh basil leaves c / n Salt to taste c / n

Direction:

1. Peel the carrots without their peel and then vicinity it in a blender or blender with a bit of the cooking water.

2. Add olive oil and salt to taste. Blend for some seconds.

3. Add the chopped sparkling basil leaves and mix again. Serve the carrot mayonnaise in a bowl and beautify with clean basil leaves and ground black pepper.

DESSERT RECIPES

Classic cinnamon rolls of Cinnabon

Servings: 12 servings

Nutrition: Carbohydrates: 117g/ Protein: 15g/ Fat: 32g

Ingredients:

- 1 1/2 sticks (12 tablespoons) unsalted butter, softened, plus more for the pan
- 1/3 cup granulated sugar
- 2 tablespoons ground cinnamon
- All-purpose flour, for dusting
- 1 batch Basic Sweet-Roll Dough, recipe follows
- 1 1/4 cups confectioners' sugar
- 4 tablespoons unsalted butter, melted
- 3 tablespoons milk
- 1/2 teaspoon vanilla extract
- Pinch of salt
- 1/2 cup whole milk
- 1 1/4 -ounce packet active dry yeast (2 1/4 teaspoons)
- 1/4 cup sugar
- 4 tablespoons unsalted butter, melted and slightly cooled, plus
- more for brushing
- 1 large egg yolk
- 1 1/2 teaspoons vanilla extract
- 2 3/4 cups all-purpose flour, plus more for dusting 3/4 teaspoon salt
- 1/2 teaspoon freshly grated nutmeg (optional)

Instructions:

1. Make the rolls: Butter a 9-by-13-inch baking dish. Whisk the sugar and cinnamon in a bowl. On a floured surface, roll out the dough right into a 10-by-18-inch rectangle. Spread the butter over the dough, leaving a 1-inch border on one of the lengthy sides. Top with the cinnamon sugar. Brush the easy border with water. Tightly roll the dough into an 18-inch log, rolling closer to the clean border; pinch the seam to seal.

2. Slip a protracted taut piece of thread or unflavored floss beneath the roll, approximately 1 half of inches from the end. Lift the terms of the thread and move over the roll, pulling tightly to cut off a piece. Repeat, cutting each 1 half inches, to make 12 rolls.

3. Cover the rolls loosely with plastic wrap and let upward thrust in a heat location till doubled in size, about 1 hour, 10 minutes.

4. Preheat the oven to 350 levels F. Uncover the rolls and bake until they spring lower back while pressed, 25 to 30 minutes. Let cool 10 mins in the pan. (You can freeze the baked rolls for up to 2 weeks. Cool absolutely before freezing, then thaw, heat up and glaze before serving.)

5. Make the glaze: Whisk the confectioners' sugar, melted butter, milk, vanilla and salt in a bowl till smooth. Drizzle over the nice and cozy rolls.

6. Warm half cup water and the milk in a saucepan over low warmness till a thermometer registers a hundred degrees F to a hundred and ten degrees F. Remove from the heat and sprinkle the yeast on top, then sprinkle with a pinch of the sugar; set aside, undisturbed, until foamy, about 5 minutes.

7. Whisk the melted butter, egg yolk and vanilla into the yeast combination till combined. In a huge bowl, whisk the flour, the final sugar, the salt and nutmeg.

8. Make a well in the center, then upload the yeast combination and stir with a wood spoon to make a thick and slightly sticky dough.

Turn out onto a floured surface and knead until smooth and elastic, about 6 minutes. Shape into a ball.

9. Brush a big bowl with butter. Add the dough, turning to coat gently with the butter. Cover with plastic wrap and permit rise at room temperature till the mixture is doubled in size, about 1 hour, 15 minutes.

10. Turn the dough out of the bowl and knead briefly to launch excess air; re-form into a ball and go back to the bowl. Lightly butter a massive piece of plastic wrap and lay it at once on the floor of the dough. Cover the bowl tightly with plastic wrap and refrigerate at least 4 hours or overnight.

Original Homemade Glazed Donuts by Krispy Kreme

Servings: 24 servings

Nutrition: Carbohydrates: 73g/ Protein: 6g/ Fat: 9g

Ingredients:

- 2 packs 1/4 ounce packages instant yeast or (4 ½ teaspoons) yeast
- 1/3 cup warm water 105-115F / 40-46C
- 1 1/2 cup milk (whole milk or low fat milk)
- 1/2 cup granulated sugar
- 1 teaspoon salt
- 2 Large eggs
- 1/3 cup (75 grams) butter or shortening, soften 5 cups all-purpose flour
- Canola oil for frying
- ½ cup butter melted
- 2 cups powdered sugar
- 2 teaspoon vanilla
- 5-7 tablespoons evaporated milk

Instructions:

1. A standing mixer, combine lukewarm water and yeast. Let it sit till dissolve for about 5 mins.

2. Meanwhile in a microwave secure medium bowl, heat milk for approximately 2 mins. Remove and permit it cool.

3. Add, milk, sugar, salt, eggs, shortening or butter and 2 cups of flour to bowl of yeast.

4. Mix for two mins at medium speed. Add the last three cups of flour and maintain mixing dough. Scraping down sides.

5. Place dough in a large greased bowl. Cover loosely with a smooth cloth and allow upward thrust in a warm, draft-free area for approximately 1 to 2 hours or till doubled.

6. Roll dough out on a floured floor to about 1/4-inch thickness.

Cut into doughnuts the usage of a donut cutter or cookie-cutter about one 1-inch and one 3 or 4-inch. Let stand for approximately 10 mins.

7. In a big saucepan, pour vegetable oil till it is at least 3 inches (or about five centimeters) high and vicinity on medium warmth till oil is 375 ranges.

8. Carefully drop doughnuts into warm oil, just a few at a time.

Fry, turning once, for about 3 minutes or till golden brown.

Drain on prepared paper towels.

9. In a microwave secure bowl melt the butter.

10. Remove and stir in powdered sugar and vanilla extract until the

whole thing comes collectively

11. Then evaporated milk (or sub water) till you have got reached favored consistency.

12. Dip doughnuts in glaze and allow it to drip at the rack.

Lady Fields Snickerdoodle cookies

Servings: 12 servings

Nutrition: Carbohydrates: 12.4g/ Protein: 1g/ Fat: 4.3g

Ingredients:

- 1/2 cup butter (1 stick, softened)
- 1/2 cup granulated sugar
- 1/3 cup brown sugar
- 1 egg
- 1/2 teaspoon vanilla
- 1 1/2 cups flour
- 1/4 teaspoon salt
- 1/2 teaspoon baking soda
- 1/4 teaspoon cream of tartar

Cinnamon Sugar for rolling:

- 2 tablespoons granulated sugar
- 1 teaspoon cinnamon

Instructions:

1. In a considerable bowl, cream together the butter and sugars with a mixer on excessive speed. Add the egg and vanilla and beat till combined.

2. In another bowl, combine the flour, salt, baking soda, and cream of tartar.

3. Pour the dry elements into the moist elements and blend well.

Chill dough inside the fridge for about an hour.

4. After dough has chilled, preheat oven to 300 degrees.

5. In a small bowl, integrate the sugar with the cinnamon for the topping.

6. Take round 2 tablespoons of the dough and roll it into a ball for every cookie. Roll it in the cinnamon/sugar aggregate and place onto a parchment coated cookie sheet. Slightly flatten each ball with the palm of your hand.

7. Bake the cookies for 12 to 14 mins and no more. The cookies won't appear done but will preserve to cook dinner after eliminated from the oven and left to sit down for a while.

Starbucks DIY Pumpkin Muffins

Servings: 15 servings

Nutrition: Carbohydrates: 24g/ Protein: 3g/ Fat: 4g

Ingredients:

- 1 1/2 cups flour
- 3/4 cup sugar
- 1 tsp baking powder
- 1 tsp baking soda
- 1/4 tsp salt
- 1 tsp pumpkin pie spice
- 1 1/2 cups pumpkin puree
- 1/4 cup butter, melted/cooled
- 1 tsp vanilla extract
- 1 egg
- 4 oz cream cheese, softened
- 1/2 tsp vanilla extract
- 1 tsp flour
- 2 tbsp sugar - 1 tsp milk

Instructions:

1. Preheat oven to 350 stages and line a muffin tray with liners or cooking spray.

2. In a large bowl, integrate the flour, sugar, baking powder, baking soda, salt, and pumpkin spice.

3. In a separate bowl, integrate the pumpkin, melted butter, vanilla extract, and egg.

4. Combine the wet mixture with the dry aggregate and stir until simply combined.

5. Fill muffin liners with batter about three/four full.

6. To make cream cheese filling: Place all substances into a bowl and integrate.

7. Using a piping bag or Ziploc bag with corner tip cut off, add a dollop of cream cheese combination to the muffin cups. *It will sink barely into batter.

8. Place muffin tray into preheated oven to bake for about 18-20 mins.

9. Remove from oven and permit to cool 2-three mins earlier than casting off from the tray.

10. Enjoy!

Classic Cheesecake from the Cheesecake Factory

Servings: 12 servings

Nutrition: Carbohydrates: 62g/ Protein: 42g/ Fat: 29g

Ingredients:

- 1 1/2 cups graham cracker crumbs
- 1/4 teaspoon ground cinnamon
- 1/3 cup unsalted butter or margarine, melted
- 4 (8 oz.) packages cream cheese, softened
- 1 1/4 cups sugar
- 1/2 cup sour cream
- 2 teaspoons vanilla extract
- 5 large eggs
- 1/2 cup sour cream
- 2 teaspoons sugar

Instructions:

1. Preheat oven to 475°F. Place a massive pan crammed with half inch water in oven.

2. Make crust: Mix graham cracker crumbs and cinnamon; add butter or margarine. Press crust onto bottom and 2/3 of the manner up a 9-inch springform pan covered with parchment.

Wrap a big piece of foil around bottom of pan. Freeze until filling is prepared.

3. Make filling: Use an electric mixer to mix cream cheese, sugar, bitter cream and vanilla. Blend until clean and creamy. Scrape down facets of bowl. Whisk eggs in a bowl; add to cream cheese aggregate. Blend just until eggs are incorporated.

4. Remove crust from freezer and pour in filling. Carefully area cheesecake into preheated water bath. Bake for 12 mins; turn oven to 350°F and bake till top of cheesecake turns golden, 50 to 60 mins. Remove cake to a wire rack to cool.

5. Make topping: Combine sour cream and sugar; unfold over cake.

Cover and refrigerate at least four hours.

Cracker Barrel's Double Fudge Coca Cola Chocolate Cake

Servings: 8 servings

Nutrition: Carbohydrates: 46g/ Protein: 2g/ Fat: 16g

Ingredients:

- 1 cup coca cola
- 1/2 cup vegetable oil
- 1/2 cup (1 stick) salted butter
- 3 heaping-ish tablespoons dark cocoa powder
- 2 cups granulated sugar
- 2 cups all-purpose flour
- 2 large eggs
- 1/2 cup buttermilk
- 1 teaspoon baking soda
- 1 teaspoon vanilla extract
- 1 stick salted butter
- 3 tablespoons dark cocoa powder
- 6 tablespoons milk
- 1 teaspoon vanilla extract
- 4 cups powdered sugar

Instructions:

1. Preheat oven to 350°F.

2. Butter and flour a 9x13 pan and set aside.

3. In the big bowl of a mixer, stir together sugar and flour and set aside.

4. In a saucepan, convey cola, oil, butter, and cocoa to a boil. Pour into the flour combination and beat on medium-low for approximately till a toothpick inserted in the middle comes out clean. Immediately upon eliminating cake from the oven, put together with frosting.

5. In a saucepan over medium heat, deliver butter, cocoa powder, and milk to simply boiling. Remove from warmth and whisk in powdered sugar and vanilla. Pour over cake and quick unfold.

Let cake cool to room temperature, then cowl and refrigerate until serving.

Melted Chili's Lava Cake

Servings: 4 servings

Nutrition: Carbohydrates: 37g/ Protein: 3g/ Fat: 0 g

Ingredients:

- 1 cup semisweet chocolate chips
- 1/2 cup butter
- 1 cup powdered sugar
- 3 eggs
- 1 egg yolk
- 1/2 teaspoon vanilla extract
- 6 Tablespoons flour
- caramel sauce, for drizzling
- vanilla ice cream
- Smuckers Chocolate Magic Shell ice cream topping, for drizzling

Instructions:

1. Preheat oven to 400 stages F.

2. In a microwave-secure bowl, integrate chocolate chips and butter. Microwave for two mins and whisk till smooth.

3. Whisk in powdered sugar until combined.

4. Add 3 eggs and 1 egg yolk, and whisk till combined.

5. Add vanilla and flour and mix again.

6. Generously spray four 1 cup oven-secure cups with cooking spray, and flippantly fill with batter.

7. Bake on a cookie sheet in the oven for 13-15 minutes until the outer edges are set and the center continues to be soft.

8. Remove from oven and permit cool for 2-three mins before inverting onto a plate drizzled with caramel sauce.

9. Top cake with a scoop of vanilla ice cream and drizzle magic shell topping on the pinnacle.

Copycat York Peppermint Patties

Ingredients:

- 4 cups of powdered sugar
- 1/3 cup of corn syrup
- 1/3 cup butter
- 4 or 5 drops of peppermint extract
- 8 ounces of dark chocolate
- 1 tablespoon of vegetable fat

Instructions:

1. Sift the sugar from the confectioners.

2. Add sugar, corn syrup, butter, and peppermint extract to a medium-sized dish. Mix till clean with a mixer.

3. The mint sweet is served in bite-sized balls. Excellent for approximately 20 mins. Press the patties with the bottom of a glass when you're geared up to dip.

4. Melt the chocolate in a double boiler and shorten. You can use alternative coconut oil or butter if you don't want to use vegetable shortening. The best effects are the shortening of vegetables. Drop in the melted chocolate the peppermint patties, turn over, and placed the dipped peppermint patties on both a Silpat mat or waxed paper to dry.

Nutrition:

Calories: 175kcal Carbohydrates: 27 g Protein: 0 g Fat: 7 g Saturated fat: 4 g Cholesterol: 7 mg Sodium: 27 mg Potassium: 67 mg Fiber: 1 g Sugar: 25 g Vitamin A: 80IU Calcium: 8 mg Iron: 1.1

Copycat Friendly's Peanut Butter Sauce

Ingredients:

- 2 tablespoons of butter
- 1 cup of heavy whipped cream (you can use half and a half) 1/2 cup corn syrup
- 1/2 cup of sugar
- 1/2 teaspoon of Salt
- 1 cup of plain smooth peanut butter is recommended 1 teaspoon of vanilla

Instructions:

Add heavy cream, corn syrup, sugar, salt, and herbal peanut butter in a medium warmth saucepan, melt butter. Continuously stir till the mixture is clear. Refrigerate the sauce, then add vanilla. Store within the fridge over the sauce.

Nutrition: Calories: 324kcal Carbohydrates: 33 g Protein: 7 g Fat: 19 g Saturated fat: 8g Sodium: 295 mg Potassium: 190 mg Fiber: 1 g Sugar: 25 g Vitamin A: 420IU Vitamin C: 0.2 mg Calcium: 27 mg Iron: 0.5 mg

Chocolate Bread Pudding Recipe

Bread pudding is a classic Christmas dessert that can be prepared with French bread, brioche, or loaf. Experiment with this recipe to give the dish your distinctive touch. This delicious chocolate bread pudding is perfect for serving along with sliced strawberries or raspberries and warm chocolate sauce.

Ingredients:

For the chocolate bread pudding

- 3 cups of cream or milk cream
- 1 cup whole milk - ½ cup of sugar
- 300 g of chocolate chips
- 8 egg yolks
- 2 eggs
- 1 loaf of French bread 500 g

For the chocolate sauce

- 1 cup of cream
- 250 g of chocolate chips

Step by step elaboration:

1. Gather the ingredients.

2. Spread a 22 x 33 cm baking sheet with butter. Preheat the oven to 180 ° C.

3. In a pot, combine the cream, milk, and sugar, and simmer, stirring until the sugar dissolves.

4. Remove the pan from the warmness. Add the chocolate chips and beat until melted.

5. Beat the egg yolks in a bowl.

6. Gradually add the mixture of cream and heat chocolate. Add the bread cut into square pieces of centimeters and stir till nicely covered. Let stand for 5 minutes, until the dough is tender.

7. Transfer the bread mixture to the prepared tray.

8. Cover with foil and bake for forty-five minutes. Remove the foil and bake for 15 minutes or till the chocolate bread pudding is prepared. Let cool on a rack.

9. In a small pot, boil a cup of cream. Remove from heat and upload the closing cups of chocolate chips and beat until melted, and the chocolate sauce is smooth.

10. Serve the chocolate bread pudding with warm chocolate sauce and crimson fruits.

Copycat Starbucks Cranberry Bliss Bar

Ingredients:

- 1 1/2 sticks of salted butter, diced - 1 1/2 cups of brown sugar, packaged
- 2 large eggs
- 3/4 teaspoon of vanilla extract 2 1/4 cups of all-purpose flour
- 1 1/2 teaspoon of baking soda - 1/4 teaspoon of Salt
- 1/8 teaspoon of cinnamon
- 1/4 cup dried cranberries, roughly chopped
- 6 ounces of white baked chocolate, roughly chopped Glaze: 1 pack, 8 oz cream cheese, softened
- 1 cup of powdered sugar
- 10 ounces of white baked chocolate, melted
- 1/2 cup of dried cranberries, chopped

Directions:

1. Oven preheats to 350 degrees F. Sprinkle with a cooking spray a 9x13 baking dish. Set apart.

2. Blondie: In a big bowl of brown sugar, they placed the melted butter. Mix and let cool for approximately 15 minutes until room temperature. Ladle butter/sugar aggregate with the paddle attachment in stand mixer dish.

3. Remove espresso and eggs, combine till it's miles incorporated. Whisk the flour, baking powder, salt, and cinnamon collectively in a medium bowl. Apply the dry elements to the wet gradually. Mix till it has just been incorporated.

4. Stir within the white chocolate and the cranberries. The batter goes to be dense; that's all right.

5. Spread the combination of batter into the baking dish prepared. Bake till a toothpick inserted within the center comes out easy for 28-30 minutes. (Make sure you don't bake too much. You don't need dry blond bars.)

6. Place on a rack of wire and cool.

7. Frosting: Whisk together the cream cheese and powdered sugar to your stand mixer or hand mixer till well mixed. Incorporate half of the molten white chocolate and comb.

8. Spread over blondies evenly. Sprinkle the closing white chocolate with cranberries and drizzle.

9. Cool the bars until they may be finished, then cut into triangles. Hold inside the fridge till ready to serve. We will preserve within the refrigerator for 2-4 days. Love! Enjoy!

Cheesecake Baileys

If you are a fan of Baileys Irish cream, then I will teach you how to prepare a delicious cheesecake with it. Surely in Ireland does not use Oreo cookies as the crust, but we are not opposed to using them either. Of course, you can use chocolate or vanilla cookies to make the crust. Let's go for the Baileys cheesecake recipe!

Ingredients:

For the crust

- 26 Oreo cookies
- 4 tablespoons melted butter Pinch of Salt

For cheesecake

- 1 kilo of cream cheese
- 1½ cups of ordinary sugar
- ¼ cup cornstarch
- 2/3 cups of Baileys Irish cream
- 1 teaspoon vanilla extract

For the Ganache

- 2/3 cups of cream or thick cream
- 2 cups of chocolate chips

Step by step elaboration:

1. Preheat the oven to 160 ° C and butter a removable mold of 20 to 23 cm. Line it with parchment paper buttered too.

2. Mix the Oreo cookies with melted butter and Salt. Distribute within the mold and set aside while preparing the filling.

3. In a considerable bowl, beat the cream cheese and sugar till the instruction is smooth and fluffy. Add the cornstarch, eggs, vanilla extract, and Irish cream Baileys.

4. Pour the preparation over the crust and place the pan on a massive baking sheet.

5. Bake the Baileys cheesecake for 80-90 minutes and then let it cool for 60 minutes in the oven. Finally, refrigerate until completely cold, for four hours or overnight.

6. When the Baileys cheesecake is prepared to serve, make the Ganache: In a small pot, warmness the cream or thick cream over low heat. Place the chocolate chips in a warmness-resistant box and pour the new cream on top. Let stand for three minutes. Then stir till there are no lumps. Refrigerate the Ganache until it is thick, 15 mins, and unfold it over the cheesecake. Let stand for 10 minutes and serve.

Chocolate Peanut Butter Pie

Ingredients:

- 2 cups wheat flour
- 1 teaspoon baking powder
- 2 teaspoons of baking soda
- 1/2 teaspoon salt
- 3/4 cup natural cocoa powder
- 2 cups refined sugar
- 2 eggs
- 1/2 cup vegetable oil
- 1 cup of milk
- 2 1/2 teaspoons vanilla extract
- 1 cup of hot coffee loaded, hot
- 1 cup creamy peanut butter
- 1/3 cup of sugar glass
- 1 teaspoon unsalted butter, softened
- 3 tablespoons whipping cream
- 2 teaspoons vanilla extract

Bitumen

- 4 cups of sugar glass
- 1/4 cup unsalted butter
- 1/2 cup natural cocoa powder
- 1 egg white
- 2 teaspoons vanilla extract
- 1 pinch of Salt
- 5 tablespoons whipping cream

Direction:

1. Preheat the oven to 180°C (350°F).

2. Grease and flour round molds of 23 centimeters.

3. Sift the flour with baking soda, baking powder, 1/2 teaspoon of salt, and three/four cups of cocoa.

4. Mix the sugar with the oil and eggs in a big bowl. Add the milk and a couple of half of the teaspoons of vanilla; stir properly. It includes sifted powders, then warm coffee; Mix till you have got a uniform dough. Pour the mixture into the 2 molds and bake for 30 minutes. Remove the desserts from the oven and cowl right away with foil, then cover with a kitchen towel. Let cool 10 minutes. Remove the cakes from the mildew and location on a cord rack. Cover once more with the aluminum and the cloth (steam is what maintains them moist). Allow them to chill thoroughly.

5. Meanwhile, put together the filling. Place the peanut butter, 1/3 cup of sugar glass, and 1 tablespoon of butter. Beat with an electric mixer until acremar. Add three tablespoons of cream and a pair of teaspoons of vanilla; blend well. Let stand at the same time as the cakes cool.

6. To put together the bitumen, area 4 cups of glass sugar, 1/four cup of butter, half cup of cocoa, egg white, 2 teaspoons of vanilla, a pinch of salt, and five tablespoons of cream in a bowl.

Beat with a highspeed electric powered mixer till you have got a creamy bitumen, approximately 2 minutes. Fill and stuff the cold cake.

Chinese Almond Cookies Recipe

Cookies with almond extract and almond in the center. It is said that the butter is what gives it the flavor, but if you wish, you can substitute it with butter or margarine.

Ingredients:

- 2 3/4 cups wheat flour
- 1 cup refined sugar
- 1/2 teaspoon of baking soda
- 1/2 teaspoon salt
- 1 cup lard
- 1 egg
- 1 teaspoon almond extract 48 almonds

How to do it:

1. Preheat the oven to 165 ° C (325 ° F).

2. Sift the flour with sugar, baking soda, and salt in a bowl. Add the butter and upload it with forks till you have a sandy mixture.

Add the egg and almond extract; blend properly.

3. Form balls 2 centimeters in diameter and set them up, separated five centimeters from every other, in ungreased baking sheets.

Place 1 almond on top of each ball and press with your finger to flatten slightly.

4. Bake at 165 ° C for 15-18 Mins. Place On Cooling Racks.

Nutrition: Calories: 82kcal Carbohydrates: 10 g Protein: 1 g Fat: 4 g Saturated fat: 2 g Cholesterol: 13 mg Sodium: 60 mg Potassium: 23 mg Fiber: 0 g Sugar: 4 g Vitamin A: 125IU Calcium: 8 mg Iron: 0.4 mg

Chocolate bread pudding

Bread pudding is a magical combination of eggs, bread, and milk, among other ingredients. It is a recipe that can take the form of sweet or savory and be served as breakfast or dessert. Bread desserts, sometimes called strata, tend to be mild and have a cream-like texture. However, there is a difference with levels, as these contain more eggs than cream. Whatever you call them, this act of transforming old bread and some essential ingredients into delicacies is lovely. This version of bread pudding carries chocolate and uses both cocoa powder and sparks.

Ingredients:

For the bread pudding

- 5 cups challah or challah bread - 1 cup whole milk - 1 cup thick cream
- ¾ cups of chocolate chips
- ½ cup of sugar - ¼ cup bitter cocoa powder
- 2 eggs - 1 tablespoon unsalted butter
- 1 teaspoon ground cinnamon
- ½ teaspoon salt - 1 teaspoon vanilla extract

For coverage

- ¼ cup of chocolate chips
- ¼ cup thick cream

Step by step elaboration:

1. Cut the bread into small cubes. Although you may use fresh food as it is, hard bread will absorb drinks a good deal better. If you operate fresh bread, toast the cubes lightly by spreading them on a baking sheet and putting them inside the oven at 180 ° C for 10 minutes.

2. In a massive bowl, mix bitter powder, sugar, Salt, floor cinnamon, thick cream, whole milk, vanilla extract, and eggs.

3. Add the bread cubes and chocolate chips and permit the mixture to stand for an hour for the bread to soak up the liquid.

4. Preheat the oven to 180 ° C. Spread a ten x 7-inch baking dish with butter and pour the bread and liquid aggregate.

5. Place the pan on a baking sheet and bake for 40 minutes or till the mixture is firm.

6. Cover by way of melting the chocolate chips within the microwave for multiple seconds and stirring the cream till smooth. Pour the topping over the chocolate bread pudding and serve warm or at room temperature.

Chocolate cake recipe

If you are dieting, treat yourself without guilt with this exquisite chocolate cake recipe. It's super easy to make, and I guarantee that everyone will love it. It has cookie dough and a lot of chocolate, both in the filling and in the decoration.

Ingredients:

For the mass

- 300 g vanilla cookies
- 70 g of butter
- For the filling
- 120 g bitter cocoa powder
- 25 cc of milk
- 1 tablespoon cornstarch
- 6 sachets of sweetener
- 20 g of gelatin without hydrated flavor
- 300 g of light cream or light cream
- 4 sachets of sweetener

To decorate

- Chocolate without sugar

Step by step elaboration:

1. Place the vanilla cookies in a meals processor and mash together with the melted butter. Mix both ingredients very well and tip over the bottom of a removable mold. Distribute well at some stage in the lowest and sides and bake at 180 ° C for 5 mins.

2. For the chocolate filling, put the milk in a pot with the bitter cocoa powder and blend with a twine whisk until it bureaucracy a cream. Add the cornstarch dissolved in water and mix till included.

3. Remove from heat and upload the sweetener sachets and unflavored gelatin formerly hydrated in water for 10 minutes and dissolved inside the microwave for one minute.

4. Incorporate thoroughly and reserve. Place the cream or liquid cream in a bowl in conjunction with the sweetener and beat till it is semi-cured. Add the chocolate cream while blending with the spatula until the entirety is adequately included and pour over the dough.

5. Chill the chocolate cake within the refrigerator for at least 2 hours and grate the unsweetened chocolate.

Peanut Butter Cheesecake

Ingredients:

- 700 g cream cheese
- 2 cups melted peanut butter
- 1 ½ cups of chocolate chips
- 1½ cups of sugar 1 cup icing sugar
- 7 tablespoons melted butter
- 10 wholemeal cookies
- 1 teaspoon vanilla extract

Step by step elaboration:

1. Place the wholemeal cookies in a plastic bag and weigh down them with a rolling pin.

2. Then vicinity the crumbs in a big bowl and add the melted butter. Mix nicely to create a species and sandblasted.

3. Place the sandblasting in a refractory mold, and compact the cookies. Reserve inside the fridge.

4. In a massive bowl, beat the cream cheese until smooth and add the sugar and vanilla extract. Mix constantly till there are not any lumps. Add the molten chocolate and combine it until a uniform mixture is obtained.

5. Pour on the idea of cookies and reserve.

6. In some other bowl, blend the melted peanut butter with the flower sugar.

7. Pour this practice over the previous aggregate and shape an even layer the usage of a knife to clean the pinnacle. Refrigerate the peanut butter cheesecake for four hours.

Chocolate Flan

Ingredients:

- For the candy
- 100 g of sugar
- For the chocolate flan
- 8 eggs
- 700 ml of milk
- 200 g dark chocolate
- 1 spoon of sugar

Step by step elaboration:

1. Place the sugar in a pot or inside the mold in which you may area the flan and put together the caramel.

2. Shell the eggs and place them in a bowl. Beat them with a few cord rods.

3. Mix the eggs with the milk, a spoonful of sugar, and the chopped and melted chocolate inside the microwave or in a water bath.

Integrate with the rods and pour the self-made chocolate flan practice into the flan over the caramel.

4. Place the mold inner a tray with water. Take to the oven and cook dinner in a water bath at 180 ° C for 40 minutes.

Mint Chocolate Brownies

If you love desserts and are looking for one to serve after dinner or a snack with a rich tea or coffee, here is the recipe for some chocolate brownies with mint to pamper you. They are delicious and straightforward to make. So if you have already prepared all the methods of brownie that we have shared in Pleasure on the plate, this can not be missed. Let's go for the recipe!

Ingredients:

For the brownie

- 180 g dark chocolate
- 1¼ cup sugar - 100 g unsalted butter
- 2/3 cup of flour 0000
- 3 eggs
- 1 tablespoon bitter cocoa powder
- ½ teaspoon vanilla extract
- ½ teaspoon salt

For the mint buttercream

- 100 g unsalted butter
- 90 g cream cheese
- 2½ cup icing sugar
- 5 drops of green dye
- 1 pinch of Salt
- 1½ teaspoon mint extract

For coverage

- 240 g dark chocolate
- 5 tablespoons unsalted butter

Step by step elaboration:

1. Preheat the oven to 180 ° C.

2. Melt the butter and the dark chocolate finely chopped in a water bath or the microwave, after which place the aggregate in a giant bowl.

3. Add the sugar and blend with a cord whisk and add the Salt, vanilla extract, sour cocoa powder, and eggs one with the aid of one.

4. Finally, add the flour incorporating it with enveloping movements. Mix thoroughly until you get a homogeneous mixture.

5. Pour the brownie instruction on a 22 x 28 cm mold formerly protected with mold paper and bake for 25 mins or until while you insert a toothpick, it comes out dry. Let cool on a rack. Place the butter reduce into small cubes in a blender and mix with the cream cheese until you get a creamy practice.

6. Add the mint and then the inexperienced edible dye. Finally, upload the icing sugar little through little. Beat at low speed till a homogeneous aggregate is achieved.

7. Distribute the mint buttercream over the bloodless brownie and cowl it with paper. Store within the refrigerator for 30 mins.

8. Melt the chocolate and butter in a water bath or inside the microwave and pour over the mint cream. Spread with a spatula and produce back to the fridge for 30 extra mins.

9. Cut the chocolate brownies with mint into squares of the scale you want and serve or refrigerate.

Blueberry Cheesecake

This blueberry cheesecake everyone likes and is very easy to prepare. Also, it has all the benefits of blueberries, among which its ability to prevent cardiovascular problems and degenerative diseases, as well as urinary infections. Even his ability to stop cancer in the initial period is attributed to him. According to the US health authority known as the Food and Drug Administration, whose acronym is FDA, blueberries are almost free of fats and sodium and provide a high content of vitamin C and fiber, which helps strengthen collagen, increase good cholesterol, fight free radicals, among other things.

Ingredients:

For the base

- 240 g of crispy sweet cookies
- 120 g butter

For the cheesecake

- 3/4 of Philadelphia cream cheese
- 180 ml of cream or milk cream
- 150 g of sugar
- 100 g of fresh blueberries
- 20 g cornstarch
- 2 eggs
- 1 egg yolk
- 1 tablespoon vanilla extract

For cover

- 150 g white chocolate

- 80 ml of cream or milk cream

Step by step elaboration:

1. Preparation of the cookie base

2. Process the cookies and blend with the melted butter till you get a paste. Place at the lowest of a removable mold 20 cm in diameter and five to 7 cm high.

3. Distribute in the course of the bottom, flatten with the again of a spoon or with the palm of your hand and reserve.

4. Filling Preparation

5. Mix the cream cheese with the sugar until there are not any clumps left. Add the yolk and eggs.

6. Mix the cornstarch with the cream or milk cream, blueberries, and vanilla extract. Turn the instruction over the dough.

7. Bake for 45-50 minutes at 170 ° C. Let cool in the oven.

8. Preparation of white chocolate cover

9. Chop the white chocolate and reserve.

10. Heat the cream or milk cream in a pot and upload the cream to the chopped white chocolate.

11. Mix and while melted, unfold at the blueberry cheesecake once cold.

Chocolate cake with chocolate bitumen

Ingredients:

For the mass

- 2 ¼ cups of flour - 2 1/3 cups of sugar
- 2/3 cup vegetable oil - ¾ cups of bitter cocoa powder
- ¾ cups of brewed coffee
- 1¼ cups of milk - 1 tablespoon alcohol vinegar
- ½ teaspoon salt - 2 teaspoons baking powder
- 1 tablespoon vanilla extract - 3 eggs
- For the chocolate bitumen
- 230g butter - 3 cups icing sugar
- 2 tablespoons cream or milk cream
- 1 teaspoon vanilla extract - ½ cup of Nutella
- Pinch of salt

Step by step elaboration:

1. To make the chocolate cake, you will first preheat the oven to 175 ° C.

2. Grease two 20 cm diameter molds with butter and cowl with baking paper.

3. Mix the milk with the alcohol vinegar and let stand for 10 minutes. Sift the flour and mix it with baking soda, salt, sugar, bitter cocoa powder, and baking powder.

4. In some other bowl, blend coffee, oil, eggs, milk with vinegar, and vanilla extract.

5. Add the liquid elements to the dry ones and mix very well with a wire whisk or a mixer for a minute at medium speed. Divide the dough into the 2 molds and bake for 40-50 mins or till a toothpick comes out completely clean.

6. Let the chocolate biscuits cool for 10 minutes inside the mold. Unmold and allow cooling on a rack.

7. To make the chocolate bitumen beat the butter until it's miles gentle and adds the chocolate and hazelnut cream. Beat until incorporated.

8. Add the icing sugar and blend. Finally, incorporate the cream, salt, and vanilla extract. Beat for a few minutes so that the filling is very mild and refrigerates.

9. Cut a chocolate cake in 1/2 and spread a layer with a bit of chocolate bitumen. Place the second one layer on pinnacle and unfold with asphalt.

10. Finally, place the other cake and unfold with chocolate bitumen; Refrigerate for 20 mins.

Shoney's Strawberry Pie with custard

The strawberry cake with custard is a delight that, if you like strawberries, you can not stop trying. In this step-by-step recipe, we will show you how to make the broken dough, how to make the custard, and of course, how to arrange the fruit to make the delicious strawberry cake.

Ingredients:

For the cake

- 160 grams of flour
- 100 grams of unsalted butter
- 50 grams of sugar glass
- 1 unit of egg yolk
- 5 milliliters of Vanilla Essence
- 30 grams of strawberry jam
- 300 grams of Strawberries

For the custard

- 400 milliliters of whole milk
- 100 grams of sugar glass
- 50 grams of cornstarch
- 1 unit of egg
- 1 group of egg yolk
- 5 milliliters of Vanilla Essence

Steps to follow to make this recipe:

1. Ready all the components for the strawberry cake.

2. In a bowl, mix flour and butter with the fingertips (cut into cubes and bloodless), until it paperwork exceptional crumbs.

3. Add the glass sugar to the combination and keep stirring along with your fingers.

4. Add the egg yolk and blend until it paperwork a tender dough is essential; add a bit water.

5. Wrap the dough in plastic wrap and refrigerate for 1 hour. If you want to make the damaged dough without gluten

6. Stretch the dough with a rolling pin, an area in the mildew, puncture the bottom with a fork, cowl with paraffin paper, add counterweight (which includes legumes) and take to the oven at 180 ° C for 20 minutes. Remove from the oven, eliminate the counterweight, leftover dough from the edges, and bake five higher mins. After that time, dissolve the strawberry jam in 1 tablespoon of water and unfold the base of the cake.

7. the egg aggregate, beat all of the time. Return the cream to the pot over medium warmness, continually stirring, while the mixture is thick, lower the heat and cook three extra minutes.

Add the cream to a bowl, cowl with plastic wrap to prevent a layer from being made.

8. Pour the custard into the mold where we have the broken dough spread with jam, unfold well. Arrange the sliced strawberries on the cream.

9. Brush the strawberries with the jam, slide the strawberry cake when it's far adequately curdled, and eat the identical day, although it may be saved refrigerated for 1 night.

DRINKS

Copycat Chick Fil A Frosted Coffee

Ingredients:

- 1 cup of dark roasted coffee beans
- 2 cups of cold water
- 4 cups of Edy's Slow Churn vanilla ice cream approx. 8
- measuring spoons

Instructions:

1. Coarse coffee beans are grinding.

2. Place ground espresso with water in a large box and permit it to steep overnight inside the refrigerator.

3. To get rid of beans, stress via a filter cheesecloth.

4. In a mixer, upload 1 cup of coffee to two cups of ice cream.

5. Run to a milkshake's consistency. Repeat for added service

Nutrition: Calories: 547kcal Carbohydrate: 62 g Protein: 9 g Fat: 29 g Saturated fat: 17g Cholesterol: 116 mg Sodium: 213 mg Potassium: 583 mg Fiber: 1 g Sugar: 56 g Vitamin A: 1110IU Vitamin C: 1.6 mg Calcium: 338 mg Iron: 0.2 mg Fiber: 56g

White Mocha Coffee

Ingredients

- ¾ cup almond milk rice or your favorite milk
- ½ cup white chocolate in sparks or cut into small pieces 1½ - 2 cups hot coffee freshly made extra strong Whipped cream to taste
- White chocolate to decorate

Instructions:

1. Place the white chocolate and milk in a small pot and soften the chocolate over low heat continuously blending so that it melts less complicated and does not burn.

2. Empty the espresso into the cups, both halfway or ¾.

3. Fill what is left over with the chocolate milk combination and decorate with whipped cream and further chocolate.

4. Serve and enjoy.

Godfather Cocktail

Ingredients:

- 1 oz Amaretto
- 2 ounces whiskey
- 2 Luxardo Cherries ice cubes

Instructions:

1. Fill a pitcher of rocks 2/three complete of ice cubes.

2. Add Amaretto and whiskey to the glass.

3. Stir well.

4. If desired, add a few drops of Luxardo cherry syrup to the glass.

Decorate with two or 3 Luxardo cherries.

Nutrition: Calories 254 kcal El Carbs: 15 sun El Protein: 1 sun El Fat: 1 sun El Saturated fat: 1 sun El Sodium: 2 mg Sugar: 13 sun Nutrition Calories 254kcal El

Olive Garden Watermelon Moscato Sangria

Ingredients:

- 750 MLS Moscato
- 6 6 oz Ginger Soft Drink
- 6 6 oz Monin watermelon syrup
- 4 4 cups ice
- 3/4 glass sliced strawberries
- 1 sliced orange

Instructions:

1. Wash and reduce the fruit into small slices.

2. Pour Moscato right into a large jug.

3. Pour Ginger Ale and watermelon syrup into a jar. Stir gently.

4. Add ice to the jar and stir gently.

5. Add slices of strawberries and oranges.

6. Serve with slices of watermelon if desired.

Nutrition: Calories 204 204 kcal El Carbs: 33 sun El Protein: 0 0 sun El Fat: 0 0 sun El Saturated fat: 0 0 sun El Cholesterol: 0 0 mg Sodium: 19 mg El Potassium: 84 mg El Fiber: 0 sun The Sugar: 26 sun El Vitamin A: 50 IU Vitamin C:22.2mg Calcium: 15 mg El Iron: 1.2 mg El Iron: 1.2 mg

Olive Garden Green Apple Sangria

Ingredients:

- 750 ml Moscato
- 6 ounces of pineapple juice
- 6 ounces of Granny Smith applesauce or apple wrinkles 8 cups of ice cream
- 1/2 cup of strawberries
- 1/2 cup of orange slices
- 1/2 cup of green apple slices

Instructions:

The chilled Moscato, pineapple juice and granny smith apple puree are mixed in a massive pitcher.

Stir till well-mixed Serve by installing a bowl many ice cubes, pour over ice.

Copycat Starbucks Hibiscus Refresher
Ingredients:

- 1 cup of sugar
- 1 cup of water
- 1 green tea bag
- 1 hibiscus tea bag
- 2 cups of water
- 1/4 cup of white grape juice
- 2 tablespoons of simple syrup or to taste
- 1/4 cup frozen berries

Instructions:

1. Combine the water and sugar in a casserole to create a easy syrup. Bring to a boil and cook for 2 minutes or till the sugar is dissolved. Remove from heat and cool earlier than use.

2. Use the 2 cups of water to brew the inexperienced and hibiscus tea. Enable five mins to steep and then allow to chill down.

3. Pour in a bottle the cooled tea, natural refrigerated syrup, and white grape juice. Delete to blend. Top with a choice of frozen berries and ice.

Copycat Olive Garden Peach Iced Tea Recipe

Ingredients:

- 1 cup of sugar
- 1 cup of water
- 2-3 freshly cut peaches
- 3 tea bags
- 6 cups of water

Instructions:

1. Put the water, sugar, and peaches in a saucepan over medium heat until they arrive at a boil. Reduce warmth to medium.

2. Crush the peach slices while stirring to dissolve the sugar. As soon because the sugar has dissolved, transfer off the burner, cowl it, and let it rest for about 30 minutes.

3. Brew tea

4. Bring the water to a boil, then turn it off and permit the tea baggage steep for five minutes.

5. Remove the tea luggage, let them cool to room temperature, then upload syrup to the tea and put it within the refrigerator.

6. Serve on ice and garnish with peach slices as desired.

Passion Fruit Lemonade Starbucks Style

Ingredients:

- 2 teabags of Tazo Passion iced tea
- 4 cups of water
- 4 cups of lemonade

Directions:

1. Heat the water to the boiling point.

2. Pour the water in a massive jug over the tea bags.

3. Let the tea luggage steep for 10 mins.

4. Remove the tea luggage.

5. Add the lemonade and let it cool in the fridge.

Nutrition: Calories: 119kcal Carbohydrates: 29 g Protein: 0 g Fat: 0 g Saturated fat: 0 g Cholesterol: 0 mg Sodium: 27 mg Sugar: 27 g Calcium: 8 mg 131. Copycat Chick-fil-A Frosted Lemonade

Ingredients:

4 cups of vanilla ice cream

1 can of frozen lemonade concentrate

1 teaspoon of lemon peel (from 1 lemon) How to do it

Stir all ingredients in a blender till smooth. Fill evenly into 4 glasses and serve immediately.

Calories: 604kcal Carbohydrate: 77 g Protein: 9 g Fat: 29 g Saturated fat: 17g Cholesterol: 116 mg Sodium: 213 mg Potassium: 525 mg Fiber: 1 g Sugar: 69 g Vitamin A: 1110IU Vitamin C: 5.4 mg Calcium: 338 mg Iron: 0.2 mg

Starbucks Horchata Frappuccino

Ingredients:

- 1 cup of water
- 1 cup of brown sugar
- 1 teaspoon of cinnamon
- 1 cup of almond milk
- You can only use 1 cup of vanilla ice cream
- 3-4 tablespoons of cinnamon dolce syrup
- 2 tablespoons of whipped cream
- 1/4 teaspoon of cinnamon

Instructions:

In a small saucepan, mix brown sugar and cinnamon. Add the water and let it cook for five mins or till the again of a spoon is full. Extract, allow the airtight container to chill and store. Recommendation for drinking Blend all substances in a blender. Disable it smoothly. Sprinkle with cinnamon and whipped cream as needed.

Nutrition: Calories: 494kcal Carbohydrates: 77 g Protein: 6 g Fat: 19 g Saturated fat: 10g Cholesterol: 64 mg Sodium: 466 mg Potassium: 300 mg Fiber: 1 g Sugar: 72 g Vitamin A: 615IU Calcium: 469 mg Iron: 2.2 mg

Screaming zombie

Ingredients:

- 4 ounces of lemon juice
- 1 tablespoon of sugar
- 3 ounces of orange juice
- 1-ounce light rum
- 1/2 oz Myers Dark Rum
- 1/2 ounce Bacardi Select Rum
- ½ ounce of grenadine

Direction:

In a pot, upload the lemon juice and sugar and blend properly. In the equal bowl (or cup) add orange juice and 1 oz. Rum. Play nicely with each other.

Half fill with ice a 16-ounce container and pour over it. Let the closing three ingredients swim with a spoon in sequence. It manner you are slowly pouring the liquid over a spoon's back, so it doesn't mix too much with the drink.

Coconut Whipped Cream Recipe

Ingredients:

- 1 can of Coconut cream or coconut milk with a good percentage of fat (about 400 ml)
- 1 tablespoon of sugar glass or other sweetener such as stevia (optional)
- 1 teaspoon vanilla essence(optional 1 teaspoon xanthan gum to thicken)
- To decorate:
- ground cinnamon (optional) - cocoa powder (optional) - Food dyes (optional)

Steps to follow to make this recipe:

1. The first step in making ready this coconut whipped cream is to accumulate all the ingredients that we're going to use. As you can see, I have brought numerous optional components in step with the taste and shade of the coconut cream you want to get, so that you can use those that paintings lovely for you. I'm going to apply a can of coconut cream, glass sugar, and vanilla essence because I like to add a touch of vanilla to the preparation. If you use a can of coconut milk, I advise you to leave it open within the fridge for a minimum 8 hours so that the fat solidifies. You could separate it more without difficulty from the liquid that remains, considering that we are most effective interested in the substantial part. Consequently, the milk Coconut has to have a good percentage of fats. If it is mild or mild, it's going to work now, not and will now not be established.

2. Then, we positioned the cream or coconut milk in a turmeric glass or hand blender, In this case, we add the glass sugar and the vanilla essence, and we start to beat at a quick speed so that it starts to mount with the accent egg whites or rod blender. It may be hit with a few manual rods, but it will take a lot longer to install it. The trick so that the vegan whipped coconut cream is nicely-mounted is to position in the fridge for some hours or 30 minutes inside the freezer before the glass of turmeric and the cream or coconut milk so that it is all freezing on the time of making it.

3. Once the coconut whipped cream is nicely assembled, we locate it in a bowl or bowl and upload the components that we like most with enveloping actions so that it does not get off, like some drops of a few food coloring to provide it another color or a pinch of cinnamon or cocoa powder to taste it, even higher, this is already going to match the consumer. But I adore it that way simplest with powdered sugar and vanilla essence. There are also individuals who add a pinch of salt and use it in salty dishes or sauces as if it had been bitter cream (adding a splash of lemon).

4. Now you just have to place the coconut whipped cream in the refrigerator and use it to enhance our cupcakes, cakes, cakes, biscuits, etc ... Here are a few ideas for you to use this lactose-loose cream rather than the traditional whipped cream in your self-made desserts.

Olive Garden Berry Sangria

This blended sangria of berry is the perfect amount of sweet and dry to please a crowd of mixed drinkers of wine. You're going to love this sangria if you love Olive Garden Berry Sangria.

Ingredients:

- 1 cup of raspberries
- 1 cup blackberries
- Halve 1 cup or a third of strawberries
- 1 cup of sweet wormwood
- 1 cup of grenadine
- 2 cups of raspberry and cranberry juice
- 1.5-liter bottle of Riunite Lambrusco
- 1/2 cup strawberry or cranberry vodka - Optional

Direction:

1. Place berries in the backside of a big gallon jug or two smaller two-quarter jugs.

2. Pour juice, wormwood, and grenadine over berries. Stir to combine.

3. Pour the Lambrusco over the juice-berry combination.

4. Add vodka in case you use to make a more potent drink.

5. Stir to combine.

6. Chill geared up to serve or put together with all pre-chilled substances.

7. Serve with berries in wine glasses.

Fireside Coffee

Ingredients:

- 2 cups of coffee mate
- 1 1/2 cups of instant coffee
- 1 1/2 cups of the instant chocolate mix like Nestle's or Hershey's 1 cup of sugar
- 2 teaspoons of cinnamon
- 1/2 teaspoon of nutmeg

Instructions:

Blend all the substances. Place into 1 cup of warm water 2 heaping teaspoons full of combination.

Nutrition: Calories: 1094kcal Carbohydrate: 198 g Protein: 10 g Fat: 30 g Saturated fat: 19 g Cholesterol: 89 mg Sodium: 297 mg Potassium: 921 mg Fiber: 5 g Sugar: 179 g Vitamin A: 855IU Vitamin C: 2.8 mg Calcium: 309 mg Iron: 3.3 mg

Copycat Olive Garden Berry Sangria

Ingredients:

- I used 750 ml red wine Merlot
- 2 cups of cranberry juice
- 1/4 cups of simple sugar syrup
- fresh berries such as strawberries, blackberries or blueberries for garnish

Direction:

Mix all components except the sparkling culmination in a huge container. Stir nicely to combine. Let the mixture relax for some hours before serving. To serve, placing ice in a glass, then clean fruit and sangria, and garnish the glass with a strawberry.

Nutrition: Calories: 147kcal Carbohydrates: 20 g Protein: 0 g Fat: 0 g Saturated fat: 0 g Cholesterol: 0 mg Sodium: 11 mg Potassium: 162 mg Fiber: 0 g Sugar: 16 g Vitamin C: 37,4 mg Calcium: 14 mg Iron: 1 mg

CONCLUSION

The most significant benefit of creating copycat recipes at domestic is due to the fact you can do anything with it. You can improve on it, do your very own twist to the method and a lot more. You can also be sure that it is safe because you're the one who is making it. Not handiest that, you can shop a ton of money due to the fact all of us know ingesting out is plenty more high-priced than making it yourself. You have little control over the substances within the meal while you devour out. You can't, of course, regulate the dish which you order because sauces, etc. Are made in advance. Now, believe having all the essential substances at domestic for a 2d to cook dinner the same dish with copycat restaurant recipes. So, when you're making a copycat eating place recipe, you can "wow" your family and guests. You're going to have them wondering you've picked up dinner from a favorite restaurant just by the usage of these recipes and saving fees as compared to dining out.

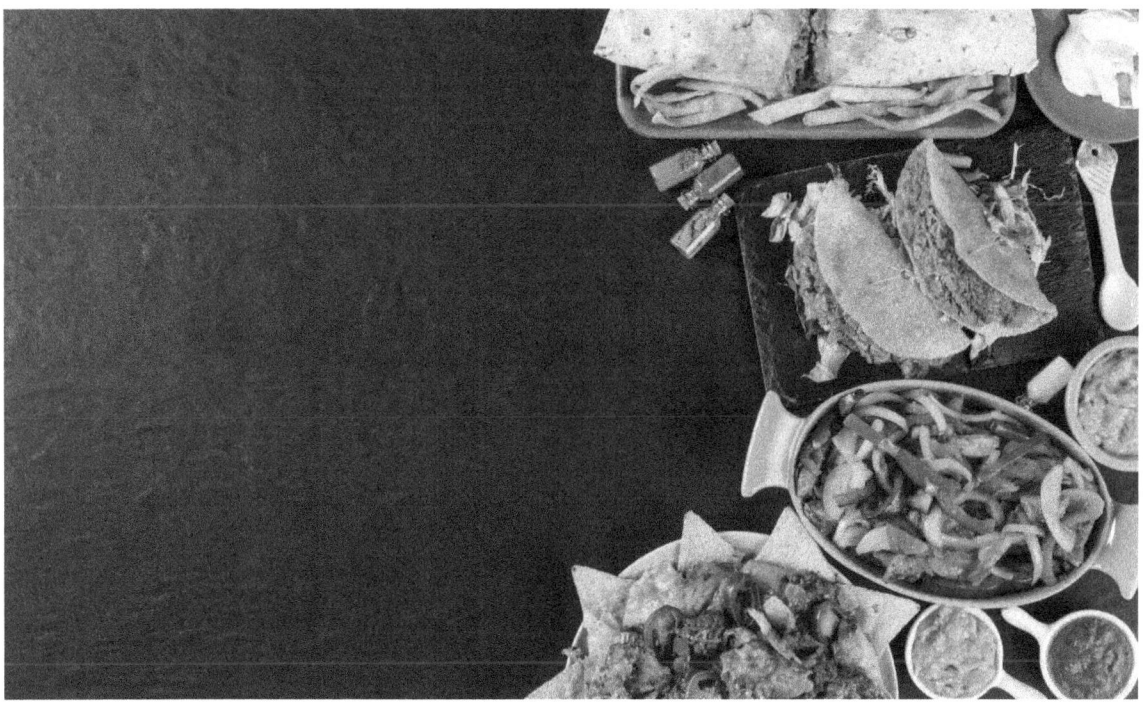

CPSIA information can be obtained
at www.ICGtesting.com
Printed in the USA
LVHW050936011220
673096LV00014B/279